Derek Bolton · Grant Gillett

The Biopsychosocial Model of Health and Disease

New Philosophical and Scientific Developments

Derek Bolton
Institute of Psychiatry, Psychology and Neuroscience, Division of Psychology & Systems Sciences
King's College London
London, UK

Grant Gillett
Bioethics Centre, Division of Health Sciences
University of Otago
Dunedin, New Zealand

https://doi.org/10.1007/978-3-030-11899-0

Preface

The problem area of this essay is set within a broad trend of increasing recognition that crossdisciplinary approaches are needed for addressing the aetiology, prevention and management of diseases. The recognition of this need goes by the name of the 'biopsychosocial model', originally proposed by the physician and psychoanalyst George Engel in a paper published in 1977. By now, some 40 years on, the model has a reasonable claim to be the overarching framework for medicine and healthcare, invoked in clinical and health educational settings the world over. Notwithstanding its popularity, however, the biopsychosocial model has come to be seen as intellectually deficient. Recent commentary sees the biopsychosocial model as being handwaving, vague, lacking scientific validity and philosophical coherence. That the aspiring overarching framework of medicine is apparently at the same time so radically flawed signals a substantial problem in the conceptual foundations of contemporary medicine and healthcare. This is the problem we address in this book. We aim to articulate a clear biopsychosocial model, drawing on Engel's original, but updating it in the light of substantial developments in the sciences and philosophy in the past few decades. While the task is focussed on the health sciences, it is set within the wider context of crossdisciplinary theory, research and problem-solving in contemporary life and human sciences.

Much evidence has emerged in the health sciences over the past few decades of psychosocial as well as biological factors being implicated in the aetiology, prognosis and clinical management of health conditions.

Typically the relative involvement of the various kinds of factor depends on the specific condition, and on stage of condition. The biopsychosocial model has stood ready to accommodate this emerging evidence, a convenient depositary, but the conceptual task of clarifying the model appropriate for this new evidence is challenging. The conceptual challenge, recognised by Engel and contemporary commentary, is that there are historically deeply entrenched assumptions—physicalism, dualism and reductionism—to the effect that only material, physical and chemical causes are real, while distinctive psychological causes and social causes are impossible or incomprehensible. Against this background, the task of theorising biopsychosocial causal interactions in health and disease is non-trivial. The result we intend however is a model that can recognise psychological and social factors as being as real and as causal as muscle strength, biochemical reactions, molecular genes or brain circuitry.

Our methodology is to work with concepts and principles worked out in the sciences, but those of a fundamental theoretical status that borders into the 'philosophical' or even 'metaphysical'. These latter terms capture the idea that core scientific theory is not just accumulated data, but rather guides empirical research and interprets its findings. Core theory has an *a priori* quality, though in the context of shifting patterns and paradigms of knowledge, not absolute. What we customarily think of as philosophy on the other hand, and science on the other, merge together in the philosophical core of scientific theory. This was so in the mechanisation of the world-picture, which combined revolutionary science with ontological statements as to the primary causal qualities of nature, assigning cognition to an immaterial status with no or inexplicable causal power. In the radical changes that have been occurring in the life and human sciences over the past few decades we find new concepts, ontology and principles of change that do not so much solve old problems as disregard the terms in which they were constructed. For example the new models in cognitive neuroscience of embodied and embedded cognition replace the old mind/body dualism and its associated problems. New biological research programmes on genetic regulatory control of cellular metabolic processes complement but exceed the physical laws governing energy exchanges in making and breaking chemical bonds, hence effortlessly, as it were, circumventing the old idea that physics and chemistry say all there is to be said about causation. In short, the conceptual apparatus needed to theorise biology as involving a distinctive form of causation, and cognitive processes as biological, as well as in interaction with the environment, natural and social—is already in the science, as work in progress, and our purpose here is only to organise some key concepts and principles into a short core theory suitable for the biopsychosocial model of health, disease and healthcare. This core theory involves new concepts and models in the health sciences, such as those implicating chronic stress as a key mechanism linking adverse psychosocial factors to poor health outcomes.

The authors have mixed disciplinary backgrounds—DB in philosophy and clinical psychology; GG in medicine, neurosurgery, philosophy and bioethics. We have written this following many years of clinical experience, research and theorising. Biopsychosocial problem-solving is trans-disciplinary—the theory breaks down traditional boundaries.

London, UK
Otago, New Zealand
January 4, 2019

Derek Bolton
Grant Gillett

Acknowledgements

This work was supported by the Wellcome Trust [grant reference 086071/Z/08/Z]. It represents independent research part funded by the National Institute for Health Research (NIHR) Biomedical Research Centre at South London and Maudsley NHS Foundation Trust and King's College London. The views expressed are those of the authors and not necessarily those of the NHS, the NIHR or the Department of Health and Social Care.

Derek Bolton

Contents

About the Authors

Derek Bolton is Professor of Philosophy and Psychopathology at the Institute of Psychiatry, Psychology and Neuroscience, King's College London. He read Moral Sciences and was awarded a Ph.D. in Philosophy at the University of Cambridge. His subsequent professional career was in clinical psychology at the Maudsley Hospital in London. He has published numerous papers in health sciences including on genetics and treatment of obsessive compulsive disorder, as well as in philosophy of psychiatry. He is the author of *An Approach to Wittgenstein's Philosophy*, Macmillan, 1979, reprinted 2013; *Mind, Meaning, and Mental Disorder: The Nature of Causal Explanation in Psychology and Psychiatry*, with Jonathan Hill, 2e, 2004, and *What Is Mental Disorder? An Essay in Philosophy, Science and Values*, 2008.

Grant Gillett is a Professor of Biomedical Ethics at the University of Otago and writes extensively on neuroethics as a sub-theme in neuro-philosophy. His professional career was in Neurosurgery and was punctuated by a D.Phil at Oxford University in philosophy of mind and metaethics. He has published in the philosophy literature on philosophy of mind and language, philosophy of medicine (particularly psychiatry), and the philosophy of medical and social sciences. He is the author of *The Mind and Its Discontents*, 2e, 2009; *Subjectivity and Being Somebody: Human Identity and Neuroethics*, 2008, and *From Aristotle to Cognitive Neuroscience*, 2018.

CHAPTER 1

The Biopsychosocial Model 40 Years On

Abstract The first chapter outlines George Engel's proposal of a new biopsychosocial model for medicine and healthcare in papers 40 years ago and reviews its current status. The model is popular and much invoked in clinical and health education settings and has claim to be the overarching framework for contemporary healthcare. On the other hand, the model has been increasingly criticised for being vague, useless, and even incoherent—clinically, scientifically and philosophically. The combination of these two points signifies something of a crisis in the conceptual foundations of medicine and healthcare. We outline some of the emerging evidence implicating psychosocial as well as biological factors in health and disease, and propose the following solution to the vagueness problem: that the scientific and clinical content of the model relates to specific conditions and stages of conditions, so that there is, for example, a biopsychosocial model of cardiovascular disease, diabetes or depression. Much the same point applies to the narrower biomedical model. However this raises the question: what is the point of having a general model? Our response is that it is needed to theorise biopsychosocial interactions in health and disease. In the light of historical prejudices against psychosocial causation deriving from physicalist reductionism and dualism, recognised by Engel and current commentators on the biopsychosocial model, this is a non-trivial task that occupies subsequent chapters.

D. Bolton and G. Gillett,
The Biopsychosocial Model of Health and Disease,
https://doi.org/10.1007/978-3-030-11899-0_1

Keywords Biomedical model · Biopsychosocial model · Philosophy of medicine · Medical models

1.1 Doing Well—But with Underlying Problems

Engel's Proposed Improvement on the Biomedical Model

In his classic paper published in 1977 George Engel proposed a new model for medicine, the biopsychosocial model, contrasted with the existing biomedical model [1]. While recognising the great advances in biomedicine, Engel argued that nevertheless the biomedical model was limited, and insufficient for many aspects of medical science and healthcare. These limitations were extensive, comprising failure to take account of the following: the person who has the illness, the person's experience of, account of and attitude towards the illness; whether the person or others in fact regard the condition as an illness; care of the patient as a person; for some conditions such as schizophrenia and diabetes, the effect of conditions of living on onset, presentation and course; and finally, the healthcare system itself also cannot be conceptualised solely in biomedical terms but rather involves social factors such as professionalisation ([1], pp. 131–135). Engel argued that a broadening of the biomedical approach, a new biopsychosocial model, was needed to take account of all these factors 'contributing to both illness and patienthood' ([1], p. 133).

The Presumed 'Overarching Framework'

In his review of a recent book on the biopsychosocial model by Nassir Ghaemi [2], in *The American Journal of Psychiatry*, Kenneth Kendler starts with the sentence: "This book is about a very important topic—the overarching conceptual framework of our field of psychiatry" ([3], p. 999).

Whether the biopsychosocial model has this status for the rest of medicine is less clear, given the prominence of biomedicine and its biomedical model. Nevertheless, 'the rest of medicine' is not one thing, and the various medical specialities differ in their relative involvement with the biological, the psychological and the social. Primary care, also known as general practice or family medicine, is well-known to be much involved in psychological and social factors, and another clear example is public health. The relevant contrast here is with biomedicine, but biomedicine is not itself a medical speciality, but a particular kind of biological science-based medicine that can be applied across medical specialities, in some more than in others. Although Engel starts his paper referring to the 'medical model', he soon switches to 'biomedical model' and this is the term he uses for the contrast with his new proposed 'biopsychosocial model'. In short it is not only psychiatry but also all the other non-biomedical aspects of medicine and its specialities that apparently require the broader biopsychosocial model.

We will review some of the health science suggesting the need for a biopsychosocial model in the next section, but first let us consider some current major trends in health, disease and healthcare that point to the same conclusion.

Engel was primarily concerned with psychosocial aspects of managing illness within hospitals, complementing the biomedical approach in hospital care. The example he discussed in detail in his 1980 'clinical applications' paper was of myocardial infarction [4]. However, it has become clear in the intervening decades that managing illnesses in hospital is a particular and expensive way of providing healthcare. Illness severe enough to require hospital admission has high burden of suffering and disability, and high costs of hospital care, including biomedical investigations and treatments. It would be better all round to prevent illness altogether, or to detect and manage it earlier to prevent worsening, and also better to provide community and social care where possible to avoid or shorten hospital admissions. Implementing this last strategy involves practical psychological and social factors, such as availability of social supports or social care. The first two strategies, primary and secondary prevention, interact with psychosocial factors such as lifestyle, social capital and health literacy.

At the same time the importance of many of the areas of neglect that Engel conveniently listed under one heading—as shortcomings of the biomedical model—have been ratcheted up by diverse trends including socio-cultural changes, economics and globalisation. The voice of the service user has gained strength from civil rights and general emancipatory social changes; rising costs of healthcare in economically developed countries have focussed minds on containing costs by service reorganisations of diverse kinds; health has become globalised in many ways, such as improving health services in economically developing countries, or in the need for international policy to manage epidemics that can now spread more rapidly worldwide.

Other trends since Engel wrote that have also broadened the focus to include more than the biomedical model have to do with changing patterns of population health. Among the greatest achievements of biomedicine have been the identification, treatment and control of infectious diseases. However, and connected, the current burden of ill health in the population now includes many conditions that are not infectious diseases and which have no available complete cure—the so-called non-infectious diseases (NCDs), sometimes also called long-term conditions (LTCs)—such as cardiovascular disease, diabetes, recurrent depression and schizophrenia. In addition, as people live longer, for many reasons including biomedical advances, the proportion of the elderly increases, especially in the absence of immigration, and care of the elderly in hospital accounts for a high proportion of healthcare costs. In short, what biomedicine is good at no longer solves a large part of the population health burden and costs, and can contribute to rising costs by keeping us alive longer (thank you at a personal level) but at great expense—to someone, especially the younger generations. What is needed to theorise all these developments is much more complicated than biomedicine or the biomedical model were ever designed for. As well as biomedicine, what is needed is a complex mix of social science, politics, economics, environmental and social epidemiology and psychology—and no doubt more scientific specialities under development.

A further development in the decades since Engel's papers that has added overwhelming weight to the case for a model that can encompass biological, psychological and social factors has been accelerating research on the causes of illness, the basis for primary prevention. The recent research, to be reviewed briefly in the next section, makes two things clear: first, that for many diseases, causes or risks are present from very early on, and second, that for many these causes or risks are combinations of biological, psychological and social. Prospective epidemiological studies suggest that risks for many major illnesses, physical and mental, start early in development, many in childhood, and that risks include *social factors* such as poverty and other forms of social exclusion, some specific *family level factors* such as neglect and abuse, and *life-style factors* such as exercise and diet. Findings on what have come to be called 'social determinants of health' were summarised and publicised for example by Michael Marmot in his 2010 Strategic Review of Health Inequalities in

England [5]. At the same time, but proceeding largely separately, there have been rapid advances in genetics. Over the past few decades many physical and mental health conditions have been found to have a genetic risk—and genetic risk starts from conception, and interacts with non-genetic factors including but not limited to psychosocial factors of the sort identified in the social epidemiological literature. In short, these sciences combined have produced a whole new dimension of the claim of the biopsychosocial model that conditions of living—as well as biological factors—may affect the onset, presentation and course of an illness.

For all these various kinds of reasons, since Engel wrote his papers some 40 years ago, the biopsychosocial model has become the orthodox overarching model for health, disease and healthcare. It is much cited and taught in healthcare trainings of all sorts and in workshops and ward rounds the world over. In simple terms it recommends to healthcare to take into account all three aspects, the biological, the psychological and the social. It is particularly useful in psychology and social work healthcare professions, and in medical practice that has to deal with the psychological and the social as much as the biomedical, primary care (family medicine) being the clearest example [6], and in-hospital medical training that emphasises the importance of a comprehensive management plan. In all these contexts the biopsychosocial model easily wins, facilitating identification and integration of different aspects of care aimed at different aspects of the patient's life, disease and management. To illustrate further good fit with much current practice, the biopsychosocial model obviously aligns with the rationale of multidisciplinary teams, and with the increasing recognition of the value of the service user's views in providing good and effective healthcare.

Given the prominent status and use of the biopsychosocial model, it is clearly of great importance that the model is clear and robust. At this point, however, there is a very large problem, because there have been increasing charges in the medical literature that in fact the biopsychosocial model—popular and accommodating as it may be—is far from being clear and robust, but is in fact deeply flawed.

But Lacks Content, Validity and Coherence

Engel's biopsychosocial model has long been criticised for having various kinds of limitation, along with suggestions for improvements (e.g. [7–9]). Increasingly, however, there have been more radical criticisms. Such radical criticisms are of two main types: first, that the model *lacks specific content*, is *too general* and *vague*; and second, that it *lacks scientific validity and philosophical coherence*. Given the popularity of the biopsychosocial model and its presumed status as overarching framework for medicine and healthcare, such radical criticisms signal significant underlying theory problems.

The first broad heading of criticism is well argued by Nassir Ghaemi, a psychiatrist at Tufts, in his 2010 book with the telling title: '*The Rise and Fall of the Biopsychosocial Model*' [2]. Ghaemi argues that the model is vague, too general, tells us nothing specific of value, hence is inefficient and sometimes distracting; it 'gives mental health professionals permission to do everything but no specific guidance to do anything' ([2], p. 82). The way Ghaemi tells the story, the biopsychosocial model arose in the context of competing general views about illness, favouring one or other of the social, the psychological/psychoanalytic and the biological. These general views—one might call them ideologies without criticism—were views of the whole domain of illness, offering general accounts, discriminating not much between kinds of case to which they applied and kinds of case to which they did not. Ghaemi interprets the biopsychosocial model as an elegant—if problematic and ultimately unviable—solution to these ideological conflicts: the unseemly turf wars could be ended, a truce could be declared, if all the participants won, if they were not really in opposition at all, but were in fact all true general accounts of illness and healthcare in all their aspects. The problem whether the cause of illness, and hence in theory its prevention and treatment, is biological, psychological or social is solved, because the answer is 'all three' ([10], p. 3; [2], ch. 6).

It has to be said that this line of thought is not apparent in Engel's main papers [1, 4]. Ghaemi does however quote a characterisation of the biopsychosocial model from another of Engel's papers consistent with presumed generality: 'all three levels, biological, psychological, and social, must be taken into account in every health care task' ([11], p. 164; [10], p. 3). This claim Ghaemi understands as meaning that the three levels 'are all, more or less equally, relevant, in all cases, at all times' ([10], p. 3). In these quotes one can see the point of the allegations that the biopsychosocial model is a slogan, too vague to be of any use. And moreover, when pinned down, more than likely just wrong, counter-evidenced exactly by the successes of biomedicine, in which biological factors alone adequately explain diseases and treatments, such as bacterial infections and anti-biotics cures. Effective biomedicine is an anomaly for any general claim to the effect that 'everything is biopsychosocial', an obvious point that warrants repetition (e.g. [2, 12]).

So, the charge is that the biopsychosocial model is vague without specific content. If, on the other hand, the model is firmed up to a very general proposition about the general relevance of all three kinds of factors, it is likely to be just false, exactly because of biomedicine. Faced with this obvious enough fact, a possible move is retreat to vagueness, but at the cost of content, as highlighted increasingly by critical commentary.

As mentioned above when illustrating the current important status or aspirations of the biopsychosocial model, Kenneth Kendler opens his review of Nassir Ghaemi's book with the statement that its topic is very important, the overarching conceptual framework of psychiatry ([3], p. 999). In his review Kendler goes on to quote Ghaemi's negative conclusion, 'The BPS model has never been a scientific model or even a philosophically coherent model. It was a slogan…' ([2], p. 213), and comments: 'While the reader may think this a little harsh…, I think he is substantially correct in this assessment' ([3], p. 999). On the other hand, Kendler ends his review with a reminder of the importance of the biopsychosocial model as a teaching tool in family medicine, concluding: 'While I agree with Ghaemi that the Biopsychosocial model has been a failure as a scientific paradigm, it probably continues to serve a useful clinical and teaching function in psychiatry and medicine' ([3], p. 999). Kendler correctly identifies the major tension here: the biopsychosocial model is a useful tool for clinical and teaching functions, but apparently lacks scientific validity and philosophical coherence.

But then probably all cannot be problem free on the teaching front either. Here is Chris McManus, Professor of Psychology and Medical Education at University College London, reviewing an earlier edited book on biopsychosocial medicine in *The Lancet* ([13], p. 2169):

> Biopsychosocial medicine's challenge is to transcend the vague, aspirational inclusivity of its name, and to create a model that truly merits being called a model, and is properly explanatory and predictive … Arm-waving and the inclusion of everything ultimately says and does little of practical consequence.

Ghaemi, Kendler and McManus all basically agree in their negative assessments of the biopsychosocial model.

Given the popularity of the biopsychosocial model, its use in teaching and the clinic, its presumed status as the overarching framework for psychiatry and perhaps for medicine generally, such authoritative negative assessment signals significant problems at the conceptual foundations.

We believe that these two kinds of charge put to the biopsychosocial model, querying its content, validity and coherence, are cogent, but can be met. What they signal is not the end of the model—witness the fact that it persists, for good reasons already indicated—but the need to rethink and reinvigorate it. The answer to the content problem, we suggest, is that the *content lies in scientific and clinical specifics*, not generalities. This is proposed in the next section, beginning with a brief review of the emerging basic and clinical science supporting the biopsychosocial model. This response to the content problem, however, immediately raises the question: if the content of the biopsychosocial model lies in specifics, what is the point of the general model? We suggest that this question relates to core scientific theory, at the place where it merges into philosophy, and is therefore here that the problem of scientific validity and philosophical coherence is to be addressed. We define this problem in Sect. 1.3, and address it in detail through subsequent chapters.

1.2 Locating the Content of the Biopsychosocial Model

Emerging Evidence of Psychosocial Causation

Just as the biomedical model is of interest because of the substantial and well-established evidence base of biomedicine, so the biopsychosocial model warrants attention insofar as there is evidence of psychological and social as well as biological factors in health and disease. There has been an accumulation of such evidence in recent decades, and before moving the main theoretical argument forwards, we pause to review some of it.

This review carries a health warning! It is uncritical and unsystematic; we have usually not distinguished strength of evidence of the studies cited below (uncontrolled to randomised controlled and replicated), nor commented on other aspects of methodological strengths (such as sampling strategies and sample size), nor on conflicting and uncertain results, nor have we employed a systematic literature search strategy. Many of the papers cited are reviews, more or less systematic. The purpose here is only to orientate the unfamiliar reader to wide range of research that has supported on-going interest in the interplay of biological, psychological and social factors in health and disease and hence the biopsychosocial model.

Over the past few decades the picture that has emerged for causes of disease onset, especially for the non-communicable diseases, also known as the LTCs, is one of complex, multifactorial causation, involving many risk factors of relatively small effect, affecting multiple outcomes. The recent research on social factors as causes or risks for poor health—the so-called 'social determinants of health'—is probably the most well-known, new face validation of the need for a broad biopsychosocial model. Among the most influential social epidemiological research programmes are the Whitehall Studies of British civil servants, led by Michael Marmot [14–16]. These longitudinal cohort studies found robust correlations between variance in incidence for a wide range of health conditions—coronary heart disease, premature mortality, some cancers, lung disease, gastrointestinal disease, depression, suicide, sickness absence, back pain and general feelings of ill-health—and civil service grade. The social gradient in health—the correlation between indices of social status and health outcomes—is now well-established; much is now known about the social determinants of health [17, 18], and something like the biopsychosocial model has to be invoked in order to comprehend it. As typically for epidemiology, most findings on the social gradient in health come from association studies only, retrospective or prospective. Establishing causation is more complex, using such as controlled cohort studies, natural experiments or animal models.

Other large research programmes have investigated associations between adverse psychosocial exposure in childhood and later health outcomes. A landmark programme is the Adverse Childhood Experiences Study (ACE Study) in the United States, carried out by Kaiser Permanente and the Centers for Disease Control and Prevention. The ACE study has demonstrated associations between adverse childhood experiences, such as physical and emotional neglect and abuse, and a large range of physical as well as mental health outcomes (e.g. [19]).

Lifestyle factors, comprising behaviours and associated beliefs, attitudes and values, have been increasingly implicated as risks, or conversely as protective factors, for a wide range of physical health conditions [14, 18]. For example risk factors for some cancers and cardiovascular disease include such as smoking, alcohol use, diet, exercise and chronic stress. Lifestyle factors can be covered under the same heading as social factors, or separately. Either way, lifestyle factors interact strongly with social context, reflecting Engel's insight that the person is essentially within a social context: diet for example, depends to some extent on choice, but also on what is available and affordable; stress—to be considered in Chapter 4—depends on individual characteristics but also on task demands and available resources.

Lifestyle and psychological factors can be distinguished: the former are behavioural, while the latter, such as beliefs, attitudes and values, are mental. At the same time they are closely linked. One reason is that psychological factors motivate lifestyle, but there is also a general linkage between our psychology and our behaviour, namely, that we respond to reality at it appears to us, at any given time, to be. We pick this up as a theoretical point in more detail later, in Chapter 3 (Sect. 3.1, heading "Mind Is Embodied"). In the present context it appears in evidence suggesting that it is not objectively measured social status but *social status as perceived*, so-called 'subjective social status' that accounts for more of the variance in health outcomes (see e.g. [20, 21]). This interesting finding becomes part of the complex jigsaw puzzle of biopsychosocial aetiology.

Over the same past few decades that evidence for psychosocial factors in health and disease has been accumulating, so also has evidence of genetic effects. For some health conditions such as Huntington's chorea, and some cancers, there are massive genetic effects, but for the majority of health conditions, the proportion of population variance attributable to genetic influence is much less than 100%, the picture being rather of relatively small effects of multiple genes, with the remaining variance attributable to non-genetic, environmental factors. Combining these broad kinds of research programmes presents a biological-psychological-social and-environmental picture, and new epigenetics is likely to help explain how the various kinds of factor interact. These issues are taken up in Chapter 3, Sect. 3.4.

Post-onset course of disease raises different causal questions: what are the processes determining course, for example, progression, stability, fluctuation or recovery? Treatment effects are a special case, assessed using a range of designs including randomised controlled trials. There has been accumulating evidence from randomised controlled treatment trials since the late 1970s of treatment effects of psychosocial interventions on some mental health conditions. Among the first was a randomised controlled trial of cognitive behaviour therapy for depression published by Beck et al. [22] showing effectiveness, but further, the same effectiveness as for anti-depressant medication. In effect this trial showed that a psychological intervention could achieve the same result as a biomedical intervention, and it paved the way for accelerating developments of tested psychological treatments for a wide range of mental health conditions and the translation of these into national health service provisions. There are complications, as always, for example, as to the extent to which psychological therapy outperforms pill placebo control, but the principle that some psychotherapies help some mental health conditions has been established (e.g. [23]).

The position is different with physical illnesses. Put strongly, there is a glaring gap in the evidence for the biopsychosocial picture as a whole, namely, absence of persuasive evidence of psychosocial treatment effects on the course of major physical illnesses. There is no clinical trial that finds effects of psychological therapy on physical illnesses such as, say, diabetes, cancers, cholera or advanced cardiovascular disease. We just wish to make the point that no psychotherapy or any other kind of psychosocial intervention turns around such disease processes once established, and this is a major apparent fact that needs to be taken into account in discussing the relative merits of the biomedical model and the broader biopsychosocial model. This is linked to the fact that for the many conditions that are managed biomedically in acute hospitals, successfully in some cases, there need be no special interest in the broader biopsychosocial model, and any advocate of the broader model has to accommodate the fact that whatever other significant roles they may have, psychosocial factors apparently make no difference to the course or treatment of major physical illnesses.

That said—and we intend it to be a big *that*—there is emerging evidence that psychosocial factors may be implicated in the prognosis of some among the very large range of medical conditions. For example: breast cancer (e.g. [24]), atopic disease, generally [25], including for asthma [26]; HIV [27–29] and musculoskeletal disorders (e.g. [30]). In addition, psychosocial factors have been implicated in outcomes of surgical procedures, for example, chronic pain [31]; lumbar and spinal surgery [32–38]; liver transplant (e.g. [39]) and coronary artery bypass (e.g. [40–42]). In addition, there is evidence for psychosocial factors in wound healing [43, 44], and extent of fatigue after traumatic brain injury [45]. Psychosocial factors have also been implicated in responses to other interventions for medical conditions, such as inpatient rehabilitation for stroke patients (e.g. [46]), and effects of hospitalisation on older patients (e.g. [47]).

Reference to psychosocial factors affecting course of medical and post-surgical conditions is not intended to be read as either conclusive or general. Many studies on this general topic are of associations only, and there are many mixed results. Hence the subtitle of this section, 'emerging evidence', and the explicit qualification of specificity to particular conditions and stages. Further, absence of reports of psychosocial effects on medical conditions, while it may suggest simply that the research has not yet been done, may also indicate that results have been negative and unpublished, and further back in the clinical research sequence, that clinicians have not seen evidence warranting case study research reports, progressing to cohort studies, and so on. This takes us back to the point made first, that some major medical conditions, such as the primary dysfunction in diabetes, or advanced cancers, or advanced cardiovascular disease, appear to be influenced exclusively by biological factors, impenetrable to psychosocial processes and interventions, and in some cases also unresponsive to biological interventions.

An old-fashioned way of making this point is to say that the mind cannot control biological processes such as abnormal cell growth. In the old dualist framework, however, the mind couldn't really control anything material, not cell growth, but not arms and legs either, so the discriminating point got lost in the metaphysics. In the new post-dualist scientific framework, to be outlined in Chapter 3, the 'mind' is not immaterial, not causally impotent, but more a matter of the central nervous system regulating some internal systems as well as the behaviour of the whole in the environment, and in these terms there are researchable differences between what the central nervous system can control and what it cannot. Extent of control may be modifiable, subject to individual differences, training and practice, but we know now that even at its best the central nervous system is not an omnipotent controller: there are places and processes that CNS signalling pathways do not reach, for example, cell growth, linked to the fact that the cells are very basic, similar in humans as in yeast; nor does the brain control the journey and final resting place of an embolus, and a long list of other biological processes and outcomes, benign or catastrophic. And this list can be contrasted with a list of biological processes and pathways that can or might have CNS involvement, as suggested by studies cited above. These issues and options only open up, however, in a new post-dualist metaphysics and biopsychological scientific paradigm, which are large themes to be addressed through the book. For now, we return to review the findings on biopsychosocial factors.

The next point to note is that, even for those physical health conditions that are unaffected by psychosocial factors, generally or at specific stages, still such factors may be relevant to clinically significant aspects of disease progression and management. These are factors such as access to treatment, participation in the recommended treatment regime, associated pain, psychological/mental health complications and health-related quality of life. Some details and literature as follows:

Access to healthcare is an obvious heading, covering diverse factors such as public health screening to ensure timely detection, health literacy, availability, accessibility and affordability of care, and quality of care—all factors heavily dependent on personal, class and state economics, associated therefore with the social gradient in health [5, 48, 49 and e.g. 50].

Acceptability of/participation in the recommended treatment regime. Psychosocial factors are associated with medication non-adherence, for example, following acute coronary syndrome [51], in haemodialysis patients [52], in youth with newly diagnosed epilepsy [53]. One systematic review of study of psychosocial factors predicting non-adherence to preventative maintenance medication therapy produced a negative result and call for more research [54].

Psychosocial factors in pain. Pain as an important phenomenon and concept spanning the biopsychosocial and will be considered further in Chapter 4. Clinical studies implicating psychosocial factors include: in chronic pain [55, 56] and in pain associated with specific conditions/sites, such as multiple sclerosis [57]; musculoskeletal pain [58, 59]; low back pain [60, 61]; spinal pain [62]; chronic prostatitis/chronic pelvic pain syndrome in men [63]; osteoarthritis [64]; cancer-related pain [65] and pain after breast cancer surgery [66].

Psychological/mental health complications of medical conditions. This is an increasingly recognised issue, with implications for quality of life (on which more below), social impairments and costs, in primary care [67], in LTCs [68] and in oncology [69, 70]. Accumulating clinical experience and research has led to a new UK NHS policy directive requiring psychological therapy services to be integrated into physical healthcare pathways [71].

Quality of life. There is a substantial literature on psychosocial factors and health-related quality of life in medical conditions, for example, in patients with haematological cancer [72]; children with myelomeningocele [73]; colorectal cancer survivors [74, 75]; myocardial infarction [76]; after hip fracture in the elderly [77]; newly diagnosed coronary artery disease patients [78]; adults with epilepsy [79], and after surgery [80]; and youth-onset diabetes myelitis [81].

Accumulating health data of the sort indicated above implicating psychosocial as well as biomedical factors, taken together, cover a large proportion of population health and health service provision in clinics and hospital beds. In other words, they are massively important, looked at in terms of population health, individual suffering, or economic costs; they are not a side-issue compared with conditions or stages of conditions that involve biological factors alone.

The psychosocial data have accumulated over the past few decades and have vindicated Engel's proposal of a new model for medicine and healthcare. Engel was ahead of the game, and the popularity of his model is explained at least partly by the fact that it appeared as a ready-made framework for accommodating the emerging evidence of psychological and social causal factors in determining health and disease.

In these terms its clear that we need a biopsychosocial model of the sort that Engel anticipated, but one that can meet the criticisms reviewed previously that the model, at least as we currently invoke it, has serious problems including lack of content and incoherence. We propose in the next section a solution to the content problem, based, as would be expected, on emerging findings implicating psychosocial as well as biological factors of the sort outlined above. As to the coherence problem, this will involve theorising the categories of 'biological', 'psychological' and 'social' in such a way that they can interact in health and disease. This theorising will occupy the rest of the book. One strand was already mentioned earlier in this section: the old dualism between mind and body is replaced by a partial and to some extent negotiable interaction between the central nervous system and other biological systems. This theory-shift will be taken up in Chapter 3, along with the proposal that the primary concept of the psychological is embodied agency, with implications for health, drawn out further in Chapter 4: a person's psychological health depends on the development of a viable enough sense of agency, while conversely, if agency is seriously compromised, such as in conditions of chronic stress, their mental health is liable to suffer, and so also, via complex biopsychosocial pathways, is their physical health.

The Scientific and Clinical Content Is in the Specifics

Let us pick up the line of argument in this chapter. The biopsychosocial model is much invoked, with claim to be the overarching framework for psychiatry and other branches of medicine such as primary care, perhaps for medicine generally. It has however been severely criticised, for being vague, without scientific or clinical content. Here is our suggested remedy: the scientific content and clinical utility of the biopsychosocial model is not to be found in general statements, *but rather is specific to particular health conditions, and, further, specific to particular stages of particular health conditions.* We provided above a brief, non-systematic, non-critical review of some of the emerging evidence of involvement of psychological and social as well as biological factors. All the evidence refers to particular health conditions or classes of conditions, and particular stages: risks for onset, post-onset course, including under treatment, adjustment and quality of life.

At the time Engel wrote there was not much evidence of causes of diseases and treatment effects, with important exceptions in the case of some major infectious diseases. But especially, compared with now, relatively little was known, though much was speculated, about the role of psychosocial factors in health and disease. Since then, in the intervening decades, there have been massive new research programmes, not only in biomedicine, but in clinical psychology, neuroscience, social epidemiology and genetics, and in treatment trials, pharmacological and psychological. Much more is now known about the causes of diseases and about possible disease mechanisms, with associated technologies for prevention, early detection and treatment. This broad evidence base has led in turn to treatment guidelines for specific conditions, to the whole apparatus of evidence-based clinical care, to be used alongside a thorough assessment of the individual case. Much of the science and clinical management is now psychological and social as well as biological. Given this situation as it is now, the scientific and clinical content of the biopsychosocial model is in the specifics, not in a 'general model'. Much the same, by the way, can be said of biomedicine and its associated biomedical model: medicine, whether biomedical or biopsychosocial, deals with complex, specific systems.

The proposal that the content problem is resolved by focussing on specifics not generality also helps explain how the problem arises. In brief, it is because the specifics are too many and too complex, that some shorthand, vague gesturing, is sometimes useful. The basic and clinical sciences of the past few decades invoke very many kinds of factors in their models: biological factors—biological systems, including neural systems and genetic mechanisms—but also psychological factors—such as temperament, personality, lifestyle, adjustment, quality of life—and also social determinants of health and disease—variants on social inclusion or exclusion—together with the implication that all these things interact over time, in the course of life and the illness, in complicated and barely understood ways. So, on occasions when the question arises, for example in clinical consultation or healthcare education systems: 'and what are the factors involved in this or that disease, or individual presentation?'—the quick answer would be: 'it's all biopsychosocial', or 'it's as the biopsychosocial model says'. The full answer is much longer, in the systemic reviews of the epidemiological and clinical sciences, treatment trials and clinical guidelines—but this full story does not fit in a ward round or clinical consultation; it more makes up years long healthcare educational training programmes. As workable compromise, the brief throwaway—'it's all biopsychosocial' could be expanded into something more informative along these lines: 'In this condition there are possibly (or probably) biological, psychological and social factors involved, in some stages, some of which have been identified, with more or less confidence, combining together in such-and-such ways, though interactive causal pathways are bound to be complex and (typically) not yet well understood—the details of what is known and hypothesised about the condition to date is in the literature/is among the topics in one of your teaching modules'.

Such an answer, and the science it refers to, is about a particular health condition, such as diabetes, or depression. In this sense there are multiple specific biopsychosocial models: a model for diabetes, depression, cardiovascular disease, schizophrenia; and so forth. Further, much depends on what stage or what aspect of a particular condition we have in mind, whether pre-onset aetiological risks for onset, or post-onset course, involving many issues including maintaining factors, treatment responses, complications, psychological adjustment and factors affecting quality of life. The factors involved in these various stages and aspects typically differ within any particular condition, and especially they differ in the relative involvement of biological, psychological and social. For example, social epidemiological studies suggest that social factors as well as biological are implicated in the aetiology of a wide range of health conditions, such as cardiovascular disease and depression, while treatment might not be so, as in surgical intervention for advanced cardiovascular disease, or pharmacological therapy for depression. This latter is typically best combined with psychological therapy, which might also be indicated to aid adjustment and recovery of quality of life following cardiovascular surgery. In short, there is need for much discrimination between what conditions we are talking about, what stages of conditions and questions of interest in each. This is the specificity and complexity of diseases and therefore of the science and its models.

We stress here that we mean no implication that particular diagnostic categories are valid once and for all, or optimal in terms of explanation or prediction. Rather, they simply represent the current consensus state of clinical practice and clinical science and are liable to revision, to subtyping or supra-typing, or to replacement altogether. The proposal is that biopsychosocial medicine, like biomedicine, is applied to specific health conditions, in terms of which the science at any one time is conducted; but identification and classification of these conditions are subject to change.

In brief, our proposal is that, while the biopsychosocial model can sometimes appear as vague hand-waving, absent any scientific or clinical content, this is because we are looking for content in the wrong place, in the general model, rather than in the epidemiological and clinical science literatures about particular conditions. This proposal, if accepted, solves the content problem.

On the other hand, that said, such a solution immediately raises a still more radical problem for the biopsychosocial model: if it's all about specifics, what is the point of having a 'general model'?!

So What's the Point of a 'General Model'?

Engel wrote about the biopsychosocial model in a way that suggested it had scientific content and clinical utility. His 1980 paper [4] was on clinical applications of the biopsychosocial model, the main example being myocardial infarction, consistent with the reasonable expectation that the model specified biopsychosocial causal pathways in particular conditions and hence could guide clinical practice. However, the position regarding what is known in the science has radically changed in the intervening decades, and now, as argued in the preceding section, the 'general model' is probably now not the place to look for causal pathways, clinical applications and treatment guidance, which are rather to be found in the health science literatures.

One possibility in the circumstances, as the evidence accumulates, is that the general model might summarise the evidence for all the health conditions, along something like the following lines: "Psychological and social factors as well as biological factors (each of these being of many different kinds) are relevant to all health conditions and all healthcare, though they vary in their relative contributions, depending on the condition and the stage of the condition, between 0-100%, or mostly between, say, 20-80% – summing to something like 100%".

However, while such a general proposition might be true, give or take some percentage points, it clearly has no or not much content, or use, in for example shaping guidance about prevention or clinical management. It is certainly less informative and useful than the full picture for a specific health condition. It is true that a general statement of the model such as the above can serve to remind us and our students to keep one's mind open to the range of biopsychosocial factors, but the treatment guidelines and the science behind them already now say this, if applicable, and there is limited gain from repeating the fact—vaguely. Used in this way, the model runs the risk of being, minimally, a bucket to throw research findings into, convenient for hand-waving purposes. As for basic scientists and clinical trialists, they investigate the causes, mechanisms and treatment of cardiovascular disease, depression, and so forth; with definitely or probably not much need or time for a 'general model'.

So what is the point of a general model? Perhaps as a theory of health and disease. But the line of thought we are pursuing is exactly that health and disease are not one thing, or two things, but each many things, depending which system within us is functioning well or poorly. Even so, the general picture still matters when the whole of health is in question, for example in estimating and projecting population health, planning and prioritising health services and research funding, on treatment, primary or secondary prevention, planning syllabuses for health education, or modelling linkages between health outcomes and outcomes in other sectors such as education, productivity or national happiness. Clinicians, patients and researchers may well be concerned with specific conditions, but for many other purposes views of the whole are required. The concept of biomedicine arose in the recognition that many effective health technologies had in common that they relied on biological factors only, notwithstanding complex biopsychosocial presentations. Such a concept then drives further lines of enquiry, investigating biological factors in other conditions. An analogous point applies to the biopsychosocial model. A related point is a need for a framework to organise accumulating research findings, to recognise emerging patterns, to identify what is known, with more or less certainty, and what is not known. This applies to specific conditions such as cardiovascular disease, or addictions, but it also applies across health conditions as a whole.

There are many purposes for a general model and accordingly many ways of constructing such a thing. We focus here on the general biopsychosocial model as *a core philosophical and scientific theory of health, disease and healthcare, which defines the foundational theoretical constructs—the ontology of the biological, the psychological and the social—and especially the causal relations within and between these domains.*

While the details of the relative roles of biological, psychological and social factors in specific health conditions, at particular stages, are matters for the health sciences, the general, or core, biopsychosocial model is more of an exercise in the philosophy of science—in this case, philosophy of biology, philosophy of mind and social theory, but especially as applied to health and disease. These philosophies are especially relevant in the present case, because there is massive historical baggage, carried in the long history of physicalism, dualism and reductionism, that makes biopsychosocial ontology and causation deeply problematic. This whole problem area needs rethinking and reconceptualising in the light of current scientific paradigms and philosophical theory.

1.3 The General Model: Biopsychosocial Ontology and Interactions

Defining the Problem

Engel was well aware of the philosophical problems involved in the shift from the biomedical model to the biopsychosocial. This is how he characterises the biomedical model ([1], p. 130):

> The biomedical model embraces both reductionism, the philosophic view that complex phenomena are ultimately derived from a single primary principle, and mind-body dualism, the doctrine that separates the mental from the somatic. Hence the reductionist primary principle is physicalistic;

> that is, it assumes that the language of chemistry and physics will ultimately suffice to explain biological phenomena.

The biomedical model so understood, as based on these philosophical views, is antithetical to any extension to a biopsychosocial model, and conversely, if the biopsychosocial model is to be viable, it has to overcome the challenges they pose. This is well recognised by thoughtful commentators on the biopsychosocial model, including those, quoted previously, who criticise the model for its hand-waving tendencies. Here is Chris McManus in his review for *The Lancet* cited previously ([13], p. 2169):

> The challenges for the Biopsychosocial Model involve reductionism, dualism, mechanism, methodology, and causality. The psychological and the sociological are ineluctably phenomena of the mind, and the reductionist challenge is how to integrate the mental with the cellular, molecular, and genetic levels at which biomedicine now works.

Ken Kendler in his review quoted earlier, goes on to identify the philosophical issues relevant to the biopsychosocial model and the work that needs to be done ([3], p. 999):

> [These are] the issues that the Biopsychosocial model at least seemed to be addressing—how to integrate the diverse etiologic factors that contribute to psychiatric illness and how to conceptualize rigorously multidimensional approaches to treatment. [There is] a range of exciting recent developments in the philosophy of science on approaches to complex biological systems, which are quite relevant to these issues… [which] examine scientific approaches to complex, nonlinear living systems and explore various models of explanatory pluralism, from DNA to mind and culture….

The importance of understanding causal interactions between kinds of factors is also highlighted by Dan Blazer in his review of Nassir Ghaemi's book [82] (p. 362):

> [There are] emerging efforts across all of medicine to integrate biological, psychological, and social factors in the exploration of the causes and outcomes of both physical and psychiatric illnesses…. These efforts are not eclectic but transdisciplinary, efforts which are leading to a much better understanding of how biological, psychological, and social factors interact through time.

Both Kendler and Blazer identify the current challenge of constructing a coherent view of causation in health and disease that can encompass biological, psychological and social factors. Kendler refers to recent philosophical developments and Blazer to emerging efforts in health sciences, both implying a historical dimension and that something new needs to happen and is happening, at a conceptual level as well as a scientific level.

Engel's characterisation of the biomedical model, a reasonable one in the 1970s, had it supposing that only the biological exists, or is alone causal in health and disease, and it exists as physics and chemistry, with the same principles or laws of causation. The ontology was flat and reductionist: nothing new grew out of the basic physics and chemistry, and any other domain with aspirations to be causal had to be ultimately reduced back to the basics. To construct an alternative to this set of assumptions it is necessary to envisage ontology and causal relations other than, and in some metaphorical sense 'above', those in physics and chemistry. Engel proposed *systems theory* for this purpose, and as we shall consider in later chapters, we think this is fundamentally the right way to go.

A systems theory approach in fact already underlies the solution to the content problem we proposed in the previous section. We proposed in Sect. 1.2, heading "The Scientific and Clinical Content Is in the Specifics", that the content is to be found in the science and clinical guidelines on specific health conditions. This is the indicated move because specific systems are distinctive, with their own distinctive functions, operating principles and vulnerabilities to dysfunction, which therefore have to be modelled separately. Healthcare science along with other systems sciences, essentially deals in specifics. This has always applied to biomedicine, which deals with particular biological systems. It also applies in psychology, which deals with particular psychological systems, such as motivation and fear, and in clinical psychological theory—for example, cognitive behaviour therapy has specific models for such as depression, obsessive-compulsive disorder and panic disorder.

The question arises then: what is the core theory linking together the various applications to specific systems? For biomedicine, in the way that Engel characterised it in the 1970s, the core theory was that biology is physics and chemistry, and biological causation is physico-chemical causation. This has changed; it is no longer true of current biomedicine; this is the topic of the next chapter. The core theory underpinning cognitive behavioural therapy, as stated by its founders Aaron Beck and colleagues [22] (p. 3) is startlingly brief, that cognitions cause affect and behaviour. However, even this brief statement of the core model does crucial work: it highlights the working assumption that intervening with cognition is the way to modify troubling emotions and behaviour, and it links together the various types of cognitive behaviour models for diverse conditions. Even in the absence of explicit theory of causation, there can be evidence of causal connection from well-designed treatment trials, but also, in this particular case there is a long and respectable history of the cognitive theory of the emotions and the philosophy of practical reason that provides conceptual familiarity for working purposes.

The contrast here is with the biopsychosocial core model: there is no long and respectable history of philosophy and science theorising causal interactions between the biological, the psychological and the social. To the contrary, the history since the beginnings of modern science in the seventeenth century consists of assumptions and arguments that psychological and social causation are impossible or even incomprehensible, that there is no distinctive biological causation either, over and above physics and chemistry. The historical background is entirely hostile to the whole idea of biopsychosocial causal pathways, and there is therefore a need for an explicit theory as to what the new idea is. It is this, we propose, that is the purpose of the general biopsychosocial model; in short, to theorise biopsychosocial causal interactions.

We review some main relevant historical background below, under the heading "Prejudicial Theory: Physicalism, Reductionism, Dualism". First, in the next section, we consider how the search for biopsychosocial theory is not only of interest to reworking a model proposed some 40 years ago, but has arisen in the health sciences themselves.

Biopsychosocial Data in Search of Theory

The emerging evidence of psychosocial causation in health and disease of the sort briefly outlined in Sect. 1.2, comes from studies using empirical methodologies that have been developed and applied substantially since Engel wrote his papers on the biopsychosocial model. Prior to these new research methods, there was little or no demonstrated evidence of psychological and social causes of physical health conditions. Their effects were not as plain—as massive—as those identified by biomedicine, as for example effects on incidence of cholera of drinking contaminated water from a particular pump, or recovery following treatment by antibiotics.

In the absence of a significant body of evidence of a causative or curative role of psychological and social factors in particular diseases, claims as to their importance were bound to have an uncertain status: were such claims meant to be general, to apply to all conditions, meant to be obvious, or based on prejudice or expert consensus—or specific to particular conditions? In the absence of much evidence, the appearance of ideology was inevitable—and this is one of the key points behind Ghaemi's critique of Engel's biopsychosocial model [2], considered previously (Sect. 1.1). However, the amount of evidence and most importantly the type of evidence bearing on these issues has changed radically in the 40 years since Engel proposed the model. We refer to use of novel statistical methodologies and associated study designs that are sensitive to multiple factors, relatively small, partial causal influences, usually called risk factors, contributing in some way to a complex nexus of causation associated with a particular outcome of interest. The development of these new methodologies was based on nineteenth-century conceptual work on the scientific demonstration of causation, and early twentieth-century work in the theory of statistical inference.

Much of the intellectual work clarifying the scientific methodology required for the determination of causes was done by J. S. Mill in his *A System of Logic* [83]. Hume [84] had seen that causality is linked to generality, that the statement 'A causes B' implies that events of type A are always followed by events of type B. This implies also that knowledge of causes enables prediction, that the next A will be B. Mill saw, however, that in practice what is observed on any one occasion is not simply an event of type A being followed by an event of type B, but this conjunction in a complex of circumstances, C. To establish a causal link between A and B the possible confounding effects of C have to be determined. This involves observing the effects of C without A, on the one hand, and A without C on the other. These principles, elucidated by Mill as the 'methods of agreement and difference', underlie our modern idea of controlled experimentation.

Robert Koch's pioneering work in microbiology in the closing decades of the nineteenth century made four postulates as methodology to determine the causal relationship between a microbe and a disease, applied to the aetiology of cholera and tuberculosis [85, 86]. Koch's postulates tapped similar principles to Mill's, including assumptions of generality and isolation of the suspected active causal ingredient—'isolation' here requiring cutting edge technology of the time.

Interestingly Koch himself recognised that there was a problem with the generality requirement, which takes us on to the next main point.

Hume, Mill and Koch supposed that causality is general—applies to 'all'. However, in practice in the lifesciences, medicine, psychology and the social sciences we rarely find universal generalisations, but rather partial ones, of the form: A is followed by B in a certain proportion of observed cases. One function of a universal generalisation is to license the simple inductive inference: the next observed A will be followed by B. In the absence of a universal generalisation, the problem is to determine the probability of the next A being followed by B, given that the proportion in the sample so far observed. This is the problem for the theory of statistical inference, developed in the first decades of the twentieth century.

The theory of statistical inference is a necessary condition of being able to detect reliable small correlations between two factors, between say amount of daily exercise and cardiovascular function at a later time. The implications of correlations being small—much less than 1 and not much above 0—is that other factors are at work, signalling the need for investigation of multiple factors associated with the particular outcome of interest. Investigation requires a group study in which each factor is each measured and their association or correlation with the outcome computed. Analysis of variance, ANOVA, is one class of statistics that can be used for such purposes: there is an outcome of interest, the so-called dependent variable, and several independent variables, hypothesised to effect it. For example, the dependent variable may be onset of cardiovascular disease by 40 years, the independent variables are individual characteristics such as weight, diet, smoking, exercise, multiple deprivation index, family history as assumed proxy for genetic vulnerability, and the results of the ANOVA will quantify the amounts of variance in outcome and hence risk attributable to these several factors, alone or in combination. Other classes of statistical analyses can be used, more or less closely related, depending for example on the nature of the variables (e.g. categorical or continuous) and on study design (e.g. cross-sectional or longitudinal). Use of such methods has become pervasive in the human sciences in the past few decades, reflecting the fact that the phenomena are complex with multiple causes; instances when a single variable completely explains a phenomenon (accounts for all or most of the variance) are rare.

Naturalistic studies of populations in the first instance establish correlations only, and further investigation is needed to establish causation, using or approximating to experimental methods of the sort elaborated by Mill and Koch. Experimental designs for establishing causation typically involve at least two groups, assumed to be identical in relevant respects—either known or suspected to affect the outcome of interest—except for one factor, the factor of interest. Differences of outcome between the two groups are then attributable to the factor of interest in accordance with Mill's method of difference. The factor of interest is often a treatment—an 'intervention'. Confidence in the assumption that the two groups are otherwise identical in relevant respects is critical in these methodologies, and there are many methods of 'matching' groups to achieve this. The philosophical justification for regarding controlled designs as the appropriate methodology for establishing causation such as treatment effects has been argued elsewhere [87]. The gold standard for maximising this confidence—the true experimental design—is taken to be randomisation, with sufficiently large numbers, such that possible confounding causal factors can be reasonably assumed to be distributed equally between the groups. Quasi-experimental designs, such as matching cohorts, can also be used, though the confidence that unknown confounders are equally matched is less. There are also 'natural experiments' (see e.g. [88]), and sometimes the background base rates absent the putative cause are safely assumed.

If we establish that a universal correlation is causal, the finding can be expressed as A causes B. Typically in the life and human sciences, correlation between factors is partial—variation in A accounts for only part of the variance in outcome B—in which case the correlation can be expressed as: A raises probability of B, in some specified degree depending on the size of the correlation. If B is a harmful outcome, such as a poor health outcome, this is often expressed: A raises risk of B, in some specified degree.

Population studies of risk factors for the onset of disease cannot use randomisation designs, plainly for ethical reasons, and are generally limited to more or less refined quasi-experimental methodology. Experimentation is left to animal studies. Treatment studies of the effect of an intervention on the course of a disease once onset can use randomisation designs—again subject to ethical constraints.

The new study designs and analytical methodologies showed effects—typically small—of psychological and social factors. The same methodology of course can show the importance of biological factors of small effect, such as genetic and epigenetic effects.

Relevant to our main theme, however, we can note that while these new study designs and statistical methodologies are well theorised, as is the determination of causes by experimental and related methods, they provide in themselves no theory of the factors indexed by the variables and no theory of causal mechanisms linking them. They can provide evidence of biopsychosocial causal connections, but no theory about them. This absence of theory is important because of the historical background of dualism and physicalist reductionism, noted at the beginning of this section (under the heading "Defining the Problem"), that would exclude any distinctive forms of biological (as opposed to physico-chemical), psychological and social causation. We review some main points of this historical background next.

Prejudicial Theory: Physicalism, Reductionism, Dualism

Engel's characterisation of the biomedical model—quoted at the beginning of this section, uses a few key technical terms: reductionism, physicalism and physicalist reductionism (Engel uses 'physicalistic'). These terms refer to complex and controversial concepts with long histories, and we will use working characterisations as follows:

Physicalism is the view that everything that exists is physical. This is an ontological statement—about what there is. It has often been combined with the corresponding statement about causation: that all causation is physical, covered by physical laws. On the assumption that chemistry is basically physics, physicalism can be expressed in terms of physics + chemistry. The contemporary philosophical literature on physicalism is substantial (for recent review see e.g. [89]). Working around physicalism is necessary to establish a biopsychosocial model and is addressed in more detail in the next chapter.

Reductionism has various meanings. In one of the senses used by Engel in his characterisation of the biomedical model, quoted at the beginning of this section, it is a scientific claim that complex phenomena have a main cause of a particular type. In the medical context, reductionism in this sense would claim that there is a main cause of one or other kind: biological (e.g. an infection or lesion), or psychological (e.g. unconscious conflicts, or maladaptive cognitive style), or social (e.g. social exclusion; labelling). There is also a philosophical or metaphysical doctrine of reductionism, deriving from physicalism, as follows:

Physicalist reductionism follows from the strong version of physicalism which has ontology and causation as all a matter of physics. It is a strict consequence for other sciences, such as chemistry, biology, psychology and social science: either they are true causal sciences, in which case they must ultimately reducible to the concepts and laws of physics; or, otherwise, they are pseudo-sciences, or at least, 'sciences' that do not deal with causation. Physicalist reductionism so understood is a philosophical or metaphysical doctrine in the sense that it is known or alleged a priori; it is not based on scientific research, but rather prejudges what there is to be discovered. Physicalist reductionism along with its roots in physicalism is taken up in the next chapter.

Physicalism has a long history, its roots lying in what historians of science refer to as the 'mechanisation of the world picture' in the seventeenth century [90–92]. This involved defining the primary qualities of nature in mathematical terms, as mass, extension and motion, covered by the few universal laws of Newtonian mechanics. The mechanisation of nature created mind–body dualism, because the thing that never did seem to be physical was immediate experience: sense-perceptions, thinking, pain and the like. Physical objects including the human body have the primary qualities, while the mind was something else, immaterial and unlocated. Physicalism and dualism are twins, one born straight after the other, combative from the start, each refuting the other, the one supported by the great edifice of modern mechanics, the other known immediately by experience, battling ever since.

It is impossible to overstate the massive influence of modern physics and its accompanying philosophy of nature on the subsequent development of western science through the eighteenth and nineteenth centuries. As sciences developed, studying apparently distinctive domains and processes, the dominant physicalism applied its stringent reductionist test: either the new aspiring science was valid as causal science, in which case it should be reducible to physics, or, it was not reducible to physics, in which case it was pseudo-science, or at best, a 'science' studying non-causes. The chemistry that emerged in the nineteenth century passed the test and joined physics. As to biology, psychology and social science, on the other hand, physicalist reductionism aided by dualism caused disunity and more or less havoc—some key points in brief as follows, to be picked up in later chapters:

Biology as we now understand it developed in the nineteenth century, drawing from previous roots in medicine, natural history and botany (see e.g. Ernst Mayr's seminal work on the history and philosophy of biology, [93]). This large, complex field, comprising many subfields, with distinctive domains, questions and methods, had an ambiguous relation with physicalism and reductionism. In some areas of biology, especially in medicine, physiology and new subspecialities such as microbiology—there was the possibility of reduction of biological phenomena as chemistry. A key development was Lavoisier's work on the relation between combustion and respiration, initiating the scientific research programme that became biochemistry. However, for other parts of the broad and diverse field of biology, reducing the phenomena of life to chemistry was not such a clear option. This applied especially to developmental embryology and evolutionary biology, which aimed to understand the formation of individual organisms and whole species, and which used explanatory concepts more akin to older, Aristotelian concepts such as form and function. Such alternative concepts, contrasted with physics and chemistry, will appear in later chapters as we develop biopsychosocial theory. Biology could embrace physicalist reductionism, or ignore it, or argue against it head on. This third option was the doctrine of 'vitalism', which posited a biological life force in addition to mechanical, or more broadly physico-chemical, forces. Vitalism is in this sense a direct response to the mechanisation of the world picture in modern science, a point made by Bechtel and Richardson [94] (p. 1051):

> Vitalism is best understood... in the context of the emergence of modern science during the sixteenth and seventeenth centuries. Mechanistic explanations of natural phenomena were extended to biological systems by Descartes and his successors. Descartes maintained that animals, and the human body, are 'automata', mechanical devices differing from artificial devices only in their degree of complexity. Vitalism developed as a contrast to this mechanistic view.

As to psychology, this new science inherited the Cartesian dualist assumptions: immaterial mind evident immediately in consciousness, and the mechanical body. Psychology struggled with the oddness of mind as its subject matter for several decades, then shifted to the other option, compatible with physicalism and reductionism, aligning psychology with physics and chemistry. This was behaviourism, and here is Watson [95] (p. 158) summarising the new approach:

> Psychology, as the behaviorist views it, is a purely objective, experimental branch of natural science which needs introspection as little as do the

> sciences of chemistry and physics. It is granted that the behaviour of animals can be investigated without appeal to consciousness… This suggested elimination of states of consciousness as proper objects of investigation in themselves will remove the barrier from psychology which exists between it and the other sciences. The findings of psychology become the functional correlates of structure and lend themselves to explanation in physico-chemical terms.

The social sciences, on the other hand, as they emerged through the nineteenth century never were going to lend themselves to comprehension in physico-chemical terms. This would be desperate business. Their subject-matter was, briefly stated, forms and processes of social organisation, which looked a very long way from physics and chemistry, further away than even psychology. As to principles of social causation, perhaps there were universal laws governing change, but equally, social systems and events appeared as specific, even unique. In short, the ontology of the natural sciences was no use to the emerging social sciences, and their methodology was of limited or questionable use. Accordingly alternative approaches developed, drawing from philosophical traditions other than physicalism, emphasising understanding and meaning, 'hermeneutics', rather than causal explanation of nature. Here is Anthony Giddens on this point [96] (pp. viii–ix):

The tradition of the Geisteswissenschaften, or the 'hermeneutic' tradition, stretches back well before Dilthey, and from the middle of the eighteenth century onwards was intertwined with, but also partly set off from, the broader stream of Idealistic philosophy. Those associated with the hermeneutic viewpoint insisted upon the differentiation of the sciences of nature from the study of man. While we can 'explain' natural occurrences in terms of the application of causal laws, human conduct is intrinsically meaningful, and has to be 'interpreted' or 'understood' in a way which has no counterpart in nature. Such an emphasis linked closely with a stress upon the centrality of history in the study of human conduct, in economic action as in other areas, because the cultural values that lend meanings to human life, it was held, are created by specific processes of social development.

To sum up, physicalist reductionism had a massive influence on the development of the biological, psychological and social sciences. It prioritised physics, subsequently physics and chemistry, as the benchmark of empirical science and causal explanation. Parts of biology measured up, as biochemistry, evolutionary biology didn't; psychology struggled; and the social sciences were so far off the mark that new views of science including alternatives to causal explanation were needed.

Against this background, deeply entrenched theory, antithetical to any distinctive forms of biological (as opposed to physico-chemical), psychological and social causation, Engel's proposal of the biopsychosocial model was audacious. It was, however, prescient, because in the intervening decades the empirical evidence has built up, as outlined in Sect. 1.2, under the heading "Emerging Evidence of Psychosocial Causation". A main virtue of the empirical, empiricist methodology of Hume and Mill, outlined in Sect. 1.3, under the heading "Biopsychosocial Data in Search of Theory", is that it can accumulate evidence of causal connections, driving the science forwards, unhindered by theoretical prejudice. The scientific methodology for determining associations and causal connections between one or more factors and a health outcome in indifferent to the nature of the factor variables involved, in particular it has no interest in whether they are called 'biological', 'psychological' or 'social'; the methodology has no interest in ontological matters at all—it cares only that the variables are measurable. Equally the empirical and statistical methodology has not much or nothing to say about causal mechanisms. Free of the historical theoretical baggage, it has been able to study relations between biological, psychological and social factors and health outcomes of interest, the upshot of which has been accumulation of evidence that psychological and social factors are at least associated with some health outcomes, physical and mental, and with some evidence of causal impact. Such free creativity is typical of empirical science. On the other hand, the downside is that we have apparently established biopsychosocial ontology and causal interactions, but so far untheorised, and—still feeling the effects of physicalist reductionism in the last few centuries of science—with perplexity and incredulity that such a thing is possible.

Theorising Biopsychosocial Interactions—Not Parallel Worlds

The proposal of biopsychosocial ontology and causal relations—under the weight of philosophical and scientific prejudice according to which psychological and social causation are impossible, even incomprehensible, and there is no distinctive biological causation either, over and above physics and chemistry—is audacious and the task of making theoretical sense of it is non-trivial.

Engel's biopsychosocial model is a very suitable heading for examining these issues. His papers certainly identified many of them, probably all that were apparent at the time he wrote them. However, Engel's model is only a heading for the major task of elucidating theory that can comprehend the paradigms and findings of the health sciences of the past few decades that invoke the full range of and interactions between biological, psychological and social factors in health and disease.

We propose to start with biology and especially its relation to physics and chemistry. It is the assumption that biology is no more than physics and chemistry that locks in the physicalist philosophy that the laws of physics and chemistry are the only causal laws. While that philosophical position remains in play, without viable alternative, it is difficult to make out any distinctive psychological or social causation and especially difficult to theorise biopsychosocial interactions. There is simply too much historical conceptual baggage in the way, variations of dualism and the disunity of the sciences.

We will be considering theory changes that have accelerated in the decades since Engel wrote. Up to the 1970s, just about everybody supposed that biology (as least as physiology) was reducible to physics and chemistry, but psychology and social sciences hardly, and so much the worse for them. In the 1970s, however, the reducibility of biology to physics became questionable, with recognition that all the 'special sciences', apart from physics/chemistry, had distinctive concepts and apparently causal explanations. However, exactly what the other sciences are sciences of, and what becomes of physicalism, dualism and reductionism, and especially how the various sciences are meant to relate to one another— all remained unclear and contested. Jerry Fodor's 1974 paper [97] had the full title 'Special Sciences (Or: The Disunity of Science as a Working Hypothesis)'. Fodor's 1997 [98] update was equally informatively titled, as 'Special Sciences: Still Autonomous After All These Years', concluding 'The world, it seems, runs in parallel, at many levels of description. You may find that perplexing…'

This parallel world view—or perhaps it should be parallel worlds plural—in which it is supposed that as well as the physico-chemical world, there is also a biological world (unless that is the same as the physico-chemical world), and a psychological world, and the social world—is certainly perplexing. It does not get much less perplexing if 'parallel world(s)' is replaced by 'many (parallel) levels of description'. Such a view however is exactly what is intellectually arrived at when forced to acknowledge, when no longer able to deny, that the biological, psychological and social sciences are now established as valid sciences including causal determinations, in some reasonable sense of 'causal', such as: can predict; when no longer able to deny this, while at the same time continuing to assume that the physico-chemical world is closed to anything other than physico-chemical causation.

This parallel worlds/levels of description approach can be applied in the health sciences, leading to the idea that psychological and social models of health and disease, as well as the biomedical, can somehow all be valid, but at different levels of description. As indicated previously in Sect. 1.1, Nassir Ghaemi argued that the biopsychosocial model has been used exactly to resolve turf wars between these various disciplines, by allowing them all to claim validity at the same time, the upshot being irredeemable vagueness and incoherence. We noted however that this thought is not prominent in Engel's papers, which philosophically relies rather on systems theory in which there is interaction between domains.

Philosophically, the parallel world(s) move, historically inevitable as it probably was, is not really coherent; what is needed rather is a more liberal view of worldly ontology and causation that can encompass not only physics and chemistry but also biological, psychological and social processes and principles of change. In any case, so far as the current sciences are concerned, and especially the health sciences, the idea of parallel causal explanations is unhelpful; rather, what is needed is theory of multifactorial interactive causation. Specifically, data of the sort reviewed in Sect. 1.2 under the heading "Emerging Evidence of Psychosocial Causation", suggesting biopsychosocial involvement in health and disease, need to be theorised in terms of biopsychosocial interactions. The quotes from Chris McManus, Ken Kendler and Dan Blazer considered at the beginning of this section, when setting up the task of the general biopsychosocial model, all refer to the need to integrate biological, psychological and social factors. Another aspect of the same point is that the various kinds of factors are found in the science to account for different proportions of the variance in health outcomes, with relative proportions of the three varying between health conditions and stages of condition. From the point of view of the science, a sentence along such lines as: 'biological, psychological and social factors (always) each severally account for 100% of the variance – at different levels of description'—is completely incomprehensible.

Finding the Right Metaphor: Evolution and Development

It is not straightforward to find the right metaphor for the relation between the biological, the psychological and the social. The most common is in terms of hierarchical levels, but it suffers from reductionist connotations that lower levels are more basic, more causal, than higher ones. Alternatively, as a transitionary move away from reductionism, appraised in the previous section, it can be interpreted as different levels of ontology and/or description running in parallel, but this makes interactions mysterious. Systemic approaches that envisage interactions are the key, major improvement, but still the metaphors struggle. One, used by Engel in his 1980 paper [4], is 'nested squares' of systemic inter-activity, from the within-body biological, outwards to self-organised activity in the external environment, including interactions with immediate conspecifics, through to complex patterns of social organisation and regulation. This 'nested' domains metaphor is not up to much either, however, insofar as it lends itself to the implicit though odd presumption that the inner domain is sorted out first, then the next grows around it, then the next around that; in effect to the idea, absurd once spelt out, that our internal biology comes first, then activity in the outside world, then activity with conspecifics. This sequencing beginning with 'first' makes no sense temporally or systemically. Internal biology, functioning in the environment, including with other biological beings, cannot be separated from one another, conceptually or temporally.

What is missing from and obscured by these two-dimensional picture metaphors of levels and nested domains is the *temporal, evolutionary and developmental, parameter*. Everything is present in the original, primitive, prototypic forms. A cell is an individual unit, separate from but essentially interacting with the environment, extracting and expending energy, including interaction with other biological entities such as viruses. Parent sea birds catch fish and put it in the mouths of developmentally immature offspring, promoting the biologically necessary energetic reactions by bringing the chemicals into close enough proximity, acting like a catalyst—unless the fish is taken away first by a bigger bird of the same or different species. All these biological-environmental-individual-within-and-between-species-interactive processes are involved from the start in the simple forms, which become ever more complex. In short, no static metaphor, whether in terms of levels or nested systems, capable of being drawn on a page, does justice to the new systems sciences, which essentially invoke dynamical interaction in present time, on the basis of co-evolution through deep time.

Developing the General Model

Evolution and development involve increasing complexity of forms, and our argument will be that these forms bring with them new causal properties. Another way of expressing this is to say that what comes into being are increasingly complex systems, and that these systems have new and distinctive causal properties. There is in particular a quantum leap at the boundary between inanimate and biological material in which new forms or systems appear that manage the physics and chemistry of the matter, specifically energy exchanges governed by physico-chemical equations. This is the argument of Chapter 2, Sect. 2.1. The biological/biomedical sciences in the last half-century have done all the work to undo the restrictive assumption that biology is only physics and chemistry and to construct instead new deep theory involving another kind of ontology, turning on dynamical forms, and causation as regulation and control. The way out of physicalist reductionism starts here—exactly at the place where physics and chemistry become biology. This is the argument of Chapter 2, Sect. 2.2.

The evolution of life forms ends up with human psychological and social phenomena. This 'ends up with', as currently understood in the science, is not a matter of logic or scientific law, but is entirely contingent—accidental. In this sense, biopsychosocial systems theory is unlike some traditional philosophical systems, which start with axioms and deduce the rest, or which elucidate natural law that covers everything. So when we move from defining key features of biology, in Chapter 2, to defining key features of psychological and hence social phenomena in Chapter 3, there is a gap, evident at the start in Sect. 3.1, one which cannot be filled in by logic or natural law, but only by contingent facts of evolution, development and change.

Human psychological and social phenomena have lives of their own—multiple distinctive modes of operation, turning on systemic concepts and principles already evident in biology, such as *form*, *organisation*, *ends*, *communication*, *rules* and *regulations*. In the evolution and development of new forms or systems, it can be said that they all share—from the start, and remaining in—the same 'ontological space/time'. This is a good way of capturing the fact that they can bump into one another and affect one another, that they causally interact, as opposed to being in parallel universes. This is to say, the ontological point is at the same time essentially a point about causal interaction. We propose defining key features of psychosocial phenomena and causation in the first sections of Chapter 3, Sects. 3.1–3.4, consistent with the key features of biology proposed in Chapter 2. With the whole biopsychosocial system in view, we return in Sect. 3.4, to the general theory of biopsychological systems, interwoven ontology and causal theory. We address the vexed issues of top-down causes, vexed from the point of view of physicalist reductionism: psychological effects on biological processes, and social effects on our biology and psychology. However, by this stage in the argument—and in the current science we intend to be tracking—the prejudicial concepts and assumptions of physicalist reductionism are nowhere to be seen. Rather, in the new approach, there are coherent core concepts and principles of causation by regulatory control, which are found already in biology, and which can elucidate in a relatively straightforward way the logic of what is traditionally regarded as top-down processing in biological, psychological and social domains. In brief, control mechanisms employ agents at the lower level, compliant with any laws that may apply at that level, but also acting as messengers from higher levels, defined by networks of relations at those higher levels.

The detailed arguments elucidating the general theory of biopsychosocial interactions are developed through the next two chapters. The fourth chapter expands on relevance to health and disease. In fact, however, the whole theory is at its core, from the start, a theory of health and disease. This is because the theory is fundamentally normative, in terms of concepts such as functioning well or badly, being well or unwell. The contrast here with physicalist reductionism is striking: the old theory makes a point of excluding any hint of normativity, with no interest in any difference between life and death or anything else related.

References

1. Engel, G. L. (1977). The need for a new medical model: A challenge for biomedicine. *Science, 196*(4286), 129–136.
2. Ghaemi, S. N. (2010). *The rise and fall of the biopsychosocial model: Reconciling art and science in psychiatry*. Baltimore, MD: Johns Hopkins University Press.
3. Kendler, K. S. (2010). [Book Review] The rise and fall of the biopsychosocial model: Reconciling art and science in psychiatry. *American*

Journal of Psychiatry, 167(8), 999–1000. https://doi.org/10.1176/appi.ajp.2010.10020268.

4. Engel, G. L. (1980). The clinical application of the biopsychosocial model. *American Journal of Psychiatry, 137*(5), 535–544.
5. Marmot, M. (2010). *Fair society, healthy lives: Strategic review of health inequalities in England post-2010.* London, UK: Department of Health.
6. Frankel, R. M., Quill, T. E., & McDaniel, S. H. (Eds.). (2003). *The biopsychosocial approach: Past, present, and future.* Rochester, NY: University of Rochester Press.
7. Sadler, J. Z., & Hulgus, Y. F. (1990). Knowing, valuing, acting: Clues to revising the biopsychosocial model. *Comprehensive Psychiatry, 31*(3), 185–195.
8. Lindau, S. T., Laumann, E. O., Levinson, W., & Waite, L. J. (2003). Synthesis of scientific disciplines in pursuit of health: The interactive biopsychosocial model. *Perspectives in Biology and Medicine, 46*(Suppl. 3), S74–S86.
9. Smith, R. C., Fortin, A. H., Dwamena, F., & Frankel, R. M. (2013). An evidence-based patient-centered method makes the biopsychosocial model scientific. *Patient Education and Counseling, 91*(3), 265–270. https://doi.org/10.1016/j.pec.2012.12.010.
10. Ghaemi, S. N. (2009). The rise and fall of the biopsychosocial model. *The British Journal of Psychiatry, 195*(1), 3–4.
11. Engel, G. L. (1978). The biopsychosocial model and the education of health professionals. *General Hospital Psychiatry, 1*(2), 156–165.
12. Davey Smith, G. (2005). The biopsychosocial approach: A note of caution. In P. D. White (Ed.), *Biopsychosocial medicine: An integrated approach to understanding illness* (pp. 77–102). New York, NY: Oxford University Press.
13. McManus, C. (2005). Engel, Engels, and the side of the angels. *The Lancet, 365*(9478), 2169–2170. https://doi.org/10.1016/S0140-6736(05)66761-X.
14. Marmot, M. (2005). Remediable or preventable social factors in the aetiology and prognosis of medical disorders. In P. D. White (Ed.), *Biopsychosocial medicine: An integrated approach to understanding illness* (pp. 39–58). New York, NY: Oxford University Press.
15. Marmot, M. (2006). Status syndrome: A challenge to medicine. *Journal of the American Medical Association, 295*(11), 1304–1307.
16. Marmot, M. G., Rose, G., Shipley, M., & Hamilton, P. J. (1978). Employment grade and coronary heart disease in British civil servants. *Journal of Epidemiology and Community Health, 32*(4), 244–249.
17. Link, B. G., & Phelan, J. (1995). Social conditions as fundamental causes of disease. *Journal of Health and Social behavior*, Special Issue, 80–94.
18. Cockerham, W. C. (2007). *Social causes of health and disease.* Cambridge: Polity Press.

19. Felitti, V. J., Anda, R. F., Nordenberg, D., Williamson, D. F., Spitz, A. M., Edwards, V., et al. (1998). Relationship of childhood abuse and household dysfunction to many of the leading causes of death in adults. The Adverse Childhood Experiences (ACE) Study. *American Journal of Preventative Medicine, 14*(4), 245–258.
20. Adler, N. E., Epel, E. S., Castellazzo, G., & Ickovics, J. R. (2000). Relationship of subjective and objective social status with psychological and physiological functioning: Preliminary data in healthy, white women. *Health Psychology, 19*(6), 586–592.
21. Singh-Manoux, A., Adler, N. E., & Marmot, M. G. (2003). Subjective social status: Its determinants and its association with measures of ill-health in the WhiteHall II study. *Social Science and Medicine, 56*(6), 1321–1333.
22. Beck, A. T., Rush, A. J., Shaw, B. F., & Emery, G. (1979). *Cognitive therapy of depression*. New York, NY: Guilford Press.
23. Hunsley, J., Elliott, K., & Therrien, Z. (2013). *The efficacy and effectiveness of psychological treatments*. Report to the Canadian Psychologial Association. https://cpa.ca/docs/File/Practice/TheEfficacyAndEffectivenessOfPsychologicalTreatments_web.pdf. Accessed 21 December 2018.
24. Falagas, M. E., Zarkadoulia, E. A., Ioannidou, E. N., Peppas, G., Christodoulou, C., & Rafailidis, P. I. (2007). The effect of psychosocial factors on breast cancer outcome: A systematic review. *Breast Cancer Research, 9*(4), R44. https://doi.org/10.1186/bcr1744.
25. Chida, Y., Hamer, M., & Steptoe, A. (2008). A bidirectional relationship between psychosocial factors and atopic disorders: A systematic review and meta-analysis. *Psychosomatic Medicine, 70*(1), 102–116.
26. Ritz, T., Meuret, A. E., Trueba, A. F., Fritzsche, A., & von Leupoldt, A. (2013). Psychosocial factors and behavioral medicine interventions in asthma. *Journal of Consulting and Clinical Psychology, 81*(2), 231–250.
27. Chida, Y., & Vedhara, K. (2009). Adverse psychosocial factors predict poorer prognosis in HIV disease: A meta-analytic review of prospective investigations. *Brain, Behavior, and Immunity, 23*(4), 434–445.
28. Ironson, G. H., & Hayward, H. (2008). Do positive psychosocial factors predict disease progression in HIV-1? A review of the evidence. *Psychosomatic Medicine, 70*(5), 546–554.
29. Langford, S. E., Ananworanich, J., & Cooper, D. A. (2007). Predictors of disease progression in HIV infection: A review. *AIDS Research and Therapy, 4*(1), 1–11.
30. Laisné, F., Lecomte, C., & Corbière, M. (2012). Biopsychosocial predictors of prognosis in musculoskeletal disorders: A systematic review of the literature (corrected and republished). *Disability and Rehabilitation, 34*(22), 1912–1941.

31. Berk, H. O. S. (2010). The biopsychosocial factors that serve as predictors of the outcome of surgical modalities for chronic pain. *Agri, 22*(3), 93–97.
32. Block, A. R., Ben-Porath, Y. S., & Marek, R. J. (2013). Psychological risk factors for poor outcome of spine surgery and spinal cord stimulator implant: A review of the literature and their assessment with the MMPI-2-RF. *The Clinical Neuropsychologist, 27*(1), 81–107.
33. Celestin, J., Edwards, R. R., & Jamison, R. N. (2009). Pretreatment psychosocial variables as predictors of outcomes following lumbar surgery and spinal cord stimulation: A systematic review and literature synthesis. *Pain Medicine, 10*(4), 639–653.
34. den Boer, J. J., Oostendorp, R. A. B., Beems, T., Munneke, M., Oerlemans, M., & Evers, A. W. M. (2006). A systematic review of bio-psychosocial risk factors for an unfavourable outcome after lumbar disc surgery. *European Spine Journal, 15*(5), 527–536.
35. Epker, J., & Block, A. R. (2001). Presurgical psychological screening in back pain patients: A review. *The Clinical Journal of Pain, 17*(3), 200–205.
36. Gaudin, D., Krafcik, B. M., Mansour, T. R., & Alnemari, A. (2017). Considerations in spinal fusion surgery for chronic lumbar pain: Psychosocial factors, rating scales, and perioperative patient education. *World Neurosurgery, 98*, 21–27.
37. Lall, M. P., & Restrepo, E. (2017). The biopsychosocial model of low back pain and patient-centered outcomes following lumbarfusion. *Orthopaedic Nursing, 36*(3), 213–221.
38. Wilhelm, M., Reiman, M., Goode, A., Richardson, W., Brown, C., Vaughn, D., et al. (2015). Psychological predictors of outcomes with lumbar spinal fusion: A systematic literature review. *Physiotherapy Research International, 22*(2), e1648.
39. Fineberg, S. K., West, A., Na, P. J., Oldham, M., Schilsky, M., Hawkins, K. A., et al. (2016). Utility of pretransplant psychological measures to predict posttransplant outcomes in liver transplant patients: A systematic review. *General Hospital Psychiatry, 40*, 4–11.
40. Pignay-Demaria, V., Lespérance, F., Demaria, R. G., Frasure-Smith, N., & Perrault, L. P. (2003). Depression and anxiety and outcomes of coronary artery bypass surgery. *The Annals of Thoracic Surgery, 75*(1), 314–321.
41. Rosenberger, P. H., Jokl, P., & Ickovics, J. (2006). Psychosocial factors and surgical outcomes: An evidence-based literature review. *Journal of the American Academy of Orthopaedic Surgeons, 14*(7), 397–405.
42. Tully, P. J., & Baker, R. A. (2012). Depression, anxiety, and cardiac morbidity outcomes after coronary artery bypass surgery: A contemporary and practical review. *Journal of Geriatric Cardiology, 9*(2), 197–208.
43. Alexander, S. J. (2013). Time to get serious about assessing—and managing—psychosocial issues associated with chronic wounds. *Current Opinion in Supportive and Palliative Care, 7*(1), 95–100.

44. Soon, K., & Acton, C. (2006). Pain-induced stress: A barrier to wound healing. *Wounds UK, 2*(4), 92–101.
45. Mollayeva, T., Kendzerska, T., Mollayeva, S., Shapiro, C. M., Colantonio, A., & Cassidy, J. D. (2014). A systematic review of fatigue in patients with traumatic brain injury: The course, predictors and consequences. *Neuroscience and Biobehavioral Reviews, 47,* 684–716.
46. Chang, E. Y., Chang, E., Cragg, S., & Cramer, S. C. (2013). Predictors of gains during inpatient rehabilitation in patients with stroke: A review. *Critical Reviews in Physical and Rehabilitation Medicine, 25*(3–4), 203–221.
47. Admi, H., Shadmi, E., Baruch, H., & Zisberg, A. (2015). From research to reality: Minimizing the effects of hospitalization on older adults. *Rambam Maimonides Medical Journal, 6*(2), e0017. https://doi.org/10.5041/RMMJ.10201.
48. Felix-Aaron, K., Moy, E., Kang, M., Patel, M., Chesley, F. D., & Clancy, C. (2005). Variation in quality of men's health care by race/ethnicity and social class. *Medical Care, 43*(3), I-72–I-81.
49. Grintsova, O., Maier, W., & Mielck, A. (2014). Inequalities in health care among patients with type 2 diabetes by individual socio-economic status (SES) and regional deprivation: A systematic literature review. *International Journal for Equity in Health, 13*(1), 43. http://www.equityhealthj.com/content/13/1/43.
50. Davidson, E., Liu, J. J., & Sheikh, A. (2010). The impact of ethnicity on asthma care. *Primary Care Respiratory Journal, 19*(3), 202–208.
51. Crawshaw, J., Auyeung, V., Norton, S., & Weinman, J. (2016). Identifying psychosocial predictors of medication non-adherence following acute coronary syndrome: A systematic review and meta-analysis. *Journal of Psychosomatic Research, 90,* 10–32.
52. Ghimire, S., Castelino, R. L., Lioufas, N. M., Peterson, G. M., & Zaidi, S. T. R. (2015). Nonadherence to medication therapy in haemodialysis patients: A systematic review. *PLoS One, 10*(12), e0144119.
53. Loiselle, K., Rausch, J. R., & Modi, A. C. (2015). Behavioral predictors of medication adherence trajectories among youth with newly diagnosed epilepsy. *Epilepsy & Behavior, 50,* 103–107.
54. Zwikker, H. E., van den Bemt, B. J. F., Vriezekolk, J. E., van den Ende, C. H. M., & Dulmen, S. (2014). Psychosocial predictors of non-adherence to chronic medication: Systematic review of longitudinal studies. *Patient Preference and Adherence, 8,* 519–563.
55. Edwards, R. R., Dworkin, R. H., Sullivan, M. D., Turk, D. C., & Wasan, A. D. (2016). The role of psychosocial processes in the development and maintenance of chronic pain. *The Journal of Pain, 17*(9), T70–T92.
56. Ong, K. S., & Keng, S. B. (2003). The biological, social, and psychological relationship between depression and chronic pain. *The Journal of Craniomandibular & Sleep Practice, 21*(4), 286–294.

57. Harrison, A. M., McCracken, L. M., Bogosian, A., & Moss-Morris, R. (2015). Towards a better understanding of MS pain: A systematic review of potentially modifiable psychosocial factors. *Journal of Psychosomatic Research, 78*(1), 12–24.
58. Mallen, C. D., Peat, G., Thomas, E., Dunn, K. M., & Croft, P. R. (2007). Prognostic factors for musculoskeletal pain in primary care: A systematic review. *British Journal of General Practice, 57*(541), 655–661.
59. Whibley, D., Martin, K. R., Lovell, K., & Jones, G. T. (2015). A systematic review of prognostic factors for distal upper limb pain. *British Journal of Pain, 9*(4), 241–255.
60. Pincus, T., Burton, A. K., Vogel, S., & Field, A. P. (2002). A systematic review of psychological factors as predictors of chronicity/disability in prospective cohorts of low back pain. *Spine, 27*(5), E109–E120.
61. Ramond-Roquin, A., Bouton, C., Bègue, C., Petit, A., Roquelaure, Y., & Huez, J. F. (2015). Psychosocial risk factors, interventions, and comorbidity in patients with non-specific low back pain in primary care: Need for comprehensive and patient-centered care. *Frontiers in Medicine, 2*(73), 1–6.
62. Campbell, P., Wynne-Jones, G., & Dunn, K. M. (2011). The influence of informal social support on risk and prognosis in spinal pain: A systematic review. *European Journal of Pain, 15*(5), 444. e1–14. https://doi.org/10.1016/j.ejpain.2010.09.011.
63. Riegel, B., Bruenahl, C. A., Ahyai, S., Bingel, U., Fisch, M., & Löwe, B. (2014). Assessing psychological factors, social aspects and psychiatric co-morbidity associated with Chronic Prostatitis/Chronic Pelvic Pain Syndrome (CP/CPPS) in men: A systematic review. *Journal of Psychosomatic Research, 77*(5), 333–350.
64. Somers, T. J., Keefe, F. J., Godiwala, N., & Hoyler, G. H. (2009). Psychosocial factors and the pain experience of osteoarthritis patients: New findings and new directions. *Current Opinion in Rheumatology, 21*(5), 501–506.
65. Novy, D. M., & Aigner, C. J. (2014). The biopsychosocial model in cancer pain. *Current Opinion in Supportive and Palliative Care, 8*(2), 117–123.
66. Schreiber, K. L., Kehlet, H., Belfer, I., & Edwards, R. R. (2014). Predicting, preventing and managing persistent pain after breast cancer surgery: The importance of psychosocial factors. *Pain, 4*(6), 445–459.
67. Von Korff, M. (2005). Fear and depression as remediable causes of disability in common medical conditions in primary care. In P. D. White (Ed.), *Biopsychosocial medicine: An integrated approach to understanding illness* (pp. 117–131). New York, NY: Oxford University Press.
68. Naylor, C., Parsonage, M., McDaid, D., Knapp, M., Fossey, M., & Galea, A. (2012). Long-term conditions and and mental health: The cost of co-morbidities. The King's Fund and Centre for Mental Health. Available at

https://www.kingsfund.org.uk/sites/default/files/field/field_publication_file/long-term-conditions-mental-health-cost-comorbidities-naylor-feb12.pdf. Accessed 21 December 2018.

69. Parle, M., Jones, B., & Maguire, P. (1996). Maladaptive coping and affective disorders among cancer patients. *Psychological Medicine, 26*(4), 735–744.
70. Cordella, M., & Poiani, A. (2004). *Behavioural Oncology: Psychological, communicative, and social dimensions.* New York, NY: Springer-Verlag.
71. NHS England & NHS Improvement. (2018). *The Improving Access to Psychological Therapies (IAPT) pathway for people with long-term physical health conditions and medically unexplained symptoms.* London, UK: NHS.
72. Allart, P., Soubeyran, P., & Cousson-Gélie, F. (2013). Are psychosocial factors associated with quality of life in patients with haematological cancer? A critical review of the literature. *Psycho-Oncology, 22*(2), 241–249.
73. Bakaniene, I., Prasauskiene, A., & Vaiciene-Magistris, N. (2016). Health-related quality of life in children with myelomeningocele: A systematic review of the literature. *Child: Care, Health and Development, 42*(5), 625–643.
74. Sales, P. M. G., Carvalho, A. F., McIntyre, R. S., Pavlidis, N., & Hyphantis, T. N. (2014). Psychosocial predictors of health outcomes in colorectal cancer: A comprehensive review. *Cancer Treatment Reviews, 40*(6), 800–809.
75. Bours, M. J. L., van der Linden, B. W. A., Winkels, R. M., van Duijnhoven, F. J., Mols, F., van Roekel, E. H., et al. (2016). Candidate predictors of health-related quality of life of colorectal cancer survivors: A systematic review. *Oncologist, 21*(4), 433–452.
76. Kang, K., Gholizadeh, L., Inglis, S. C., & Han, H. R. (2017). Correlates of health-related quality of life in patients with myocardial infarction: A literature review. *International Journal of Nursing Studies, 73,* 1–16.
77. Peeters, C. M. M., Visser, E., Van de Ree, C. L. P., Gosens, T., Den Oudsten, B. L., & De Vries, J. (2016). Quality of life after hip fracture in the elderly: A systematic literature review. *Injury, 47*(7), 1369–1382.
78. Pragodpol, P., & Ryan, C. (2013). Critical review of factors predicting health-related quality of life in newly diagnosed coronary artery disease patients. *Journal of Cardiovascular Nursing, 28*(3), 277–284.
79. Taylor, R. S., Sander, J. W., Taylor, R. J., & Baker, G. A. (2011). Predictors of health-related quality of life and costs in adults with epilepsy: A systematic review. *Epilepsia, 52*(12), 2168–2180.
80. Seiam, A. H. R., Dhaliwal, H., & Wiebe, S. (2011). Determinants of quality of life after epilepsy surgery: Systematic review and evidence summary. *Epilepsy & Behavior, 21*(4), 441–445.
81. Walders-Abramson, N. (2014). Depression and quality of life in youth-onset type 2 diabetes mellitus. *Current Diabetes Reports, 14*(1), 449. https://doi.org/10.1007/s11892-013-0449-x.

82. Blazer, D. (2010). [Book Review] The rise and fall of the biopsychosocial model: Reconciling art and science in psychiatry. *The International Journal of Psychiatry in Medicine, 40*(3), 361–362. https://doi.org/10.2190/PM.40.3.j.
83. Mill, J. S. (1843). *A system of logic*. London: John W. Parker.
84. Hume, D. (1902). *An enquiry concerning human understanding* (L. A. Selby-Bigge, Ed.). Oxford: Oxford University Press (Original work published 1777).
85. Koch, R. (1890). Uber bacteriologische forschung. *Deutsche Medizinische Wochenschrift, 16*, 756–757.
86. Evans, A. (1976). Causation and disease: The Henle-Koch postulates revisited. *The Yale Journal of Biology and Medicine, 49*, 175–195.
87. Bolton, D. (2008). The epistemology of randomized, controlled trials and application in psychiatry. *Philosophy, Psychiatry & Psychology, 15*(2), 159–165.
88. Rutter, M. (2000). Psychosocial influences: Critiques, findings, and research needs. *Development and Psychopathology, 12*(3), 375–405. https://doi.org/10.1017/S0954579400003072.
89. Stoljar, D. (2015)., "Physicalism", *The Stanford Encyclopedia of Philosophy* (Winter 2017 Edition), Edward N. Zalta (ed.), URL = <https://plato.stanford.edu/archives/win2017/entries/physicalism/>. Accessed 12/21/2018.
90. Burtt, E. A. (1932). *The metaphysical foundations of modern physical sciences*. London: Routledge and Kegan Paul.
91. Dijksterhuis, E. J. (1961). *The mechanization of the world picture* (C. Dikshoorn, Trans.). Oxford: Oxford University Press.
92. Koyré, A. (1968). *Metaphysics and measurement: Essays in the scientific revolution*. London: Chapman and Hall.
93. Mayr, E. (1982). *The growth of biological thought: Diversity, evolution, and inheritance*. Cambridge, MA: Harvard University Press.
94. Bechtel, W., & Richardson, R. C. (2005). Vitalism. In E. Craig (Ed.), *The shorter Routledge encyclopedia of philosophy* (p. 1051). Oxford: Routledge.
95. Watson, J. B. (1913). Psychology as the behaviorist views it. *Psychological Review, 20*(2), 158–177.
96. Giddens, A. (2005). *Introduction to the protestant ethic and the spirit of capitalism, by Max Weber* (T. Parsons, Trans.). London: Routledge.
97. Fodor, J. (1974). Special sciences (Or: The disunity of science as a working hypothesis). *Synthese, 28*(2), 97–115.
98. Fodor, J. (1997). Special sciences: Still autonomous after all these years. *Philosophical Perspectives, 11*, 149–163.

CHAPTER 2

Biology Involves Regulatory Control of Physical–Chemical Energetic Processes

Abstract As Engel saw, we will never make sense of psychosocial factors and their influence on health and disease while there is an underlying assumption that only physical causes are real. We believe the place to unpick this assumption is in biology and biomedicine itself, especially in the relation between biological processes and physics and chemistry. Ernst Schrödinger's insight that biological processes run locally counter to the general direction of the second law of thermodynamics is now mainstream biophysics, as is his proposal that this is originally achieved by genes exercising information-based regulatory control of energetic processes. Information-based regulatory control mechanisms are a new and distinctive form of causation compared with conformity to the energy equations of physics and chemistry, most clearly evident in the fact that they can break down. This serves to argue against physicalism and is consistent with recent innovations in the philosophy of causation. The new concepts and principles of regulatory control apply in biology, but they also run through the psychological and social domains. This enables a more unified science, and one that has foundational differences between life and death, health and illness.

Keywords Biological causation · Biopsychosocial causation · Physicalism · Reductionism

D. Bolton and G. Gillett,
The Biopsychosocial Model of Health and Disease,
https://doi.org/10.1007/978-3-030-11899-0_2

2.1 The New Biology/Biomedicine

Life vs. The Second Law of Thermodynamics

In the mid-twentieth century Erwin Schrödinger saw that from the point of view of physics living systems can be conceptualised as local areas in which, contrary to the general direction in the universe, entropy decreases, order increases [1]. Living systems make energy differences, extracting energy from the environment, using this to maintain their difference and to function, for example to obtain more energy. Schrödinger's idea was taken up by von Bertalanffy in his *General System Theory* [2], and is now mainstream life science, at the cutting edge of understanding how biology relates to physics and chemistry, conceptually and in the appearance of life on Earth. Here is the biophysicist Nick Lane in his recent popular book *The Vital Question* [3] (pp. 21–22):

> Ironically, the modern era of molecular biology, and all the extraordinary DNA technology that it entails, arguably began with a physicist, specifically with the publication of Erwin Schrödinger's book What is Life? in 1944. Schrödinger made two key points: first, that life somehow resists the universal tendency to decay, the increasing entropy (disorder) that is stipulated by the second law of thermodynamics;…

The second point is that the key to how life does this is: *genes* and genetic information. We pick this up later, but first, more on the physics.

Energy Production and Control in Cells

Rolling entropy back—locally and definitely temporarily—is bound to involve a great deal of physics. Lane vividly explains energy production processes deep inside the cell; here are some selections [3] (pp. 69–71):

> You are at the thermodynamic epicentre of the cell, the site of cellular respiration, deep within the mitochondria. Hydrogen is being stripped from the molecular remains of your food, and passed into the fast and largest of [the] giant respiratory complexes… Electrons are separated from protons and fed into this vast complex, sucked in at one end and spat out of the other, all the way over there, deep in the membrane itself… The electrical current animates everything here… Your 40 trillion cells contain at least

> a quadrillion mitochondria, with a combined convoluted surface area of about 14,000 square metres; about 4 football fields. Their job is to pump protons, and together they pump more than 10^{21} of them… *every second.*

The key points for our present purpose are first, that biological organisms exploit physics to extract energy for functioning, and second, picked up in the next section, that their doing this depends not only and essentially on the physics but also on *massive organisational and regulatory mechanisms.*

Regulatory Control by Genetic Information

Questions about how living processes accomplish the feat or resisting entropy, at least temporarily until they return to dust, and how they persist nevertheless by making replicas of themselves—all turn out to involve *regulation* and *control, information* and *coding*. Here is Nick Lane on Schrödinger's second key point, continuing from the quote above [3] (p. 22):

> And second, that the trick to life's local evasion of entropy lies in the genes. He proposed that the genetic material is an aperiodic crystal, which does not have a strictly repeating structure, hence could act as a code-script – reputedly the first use of the term in the biological literature… Within a frenzied decade, Crick and Watson had inferred the crystal structure of DNA itself. In their second *Nature* paper of 1953, they wrote: 'it therefore seems likely that the precise sequence of the bases is the code which carries the genetical information'. That sentence is the basis of modern biology. Today biology is information, genomic sequences are laid out in silico, and life is defined in terms of information transfer.

Biological organisms use information transfer to control energy transfer. Physical and chemical processes involve energy transfers covered by mathematical energy equations, but in biological organisms the physical and chemical processes not only happen, but can only happen in the right place at the right time in the right degree, if there are mechanisms that control and regulate them in a way appropriate to bringing about a particular function. These mechanisms also conform to the physico-chemical energy equations, they never violate them, but they are not fully explained by them, rather their full explanation has to invoke concepts of information-based regulatory control, and typically involve *form*, or *structure*. Control systems assemble, organise, up- and down-regulate physico-chemical energetic processes. A control system has to be sensitive to physico-chemical processes and to other control systems, depending on their state, if they are to tend towards end states of the whole. This reactive and interactive sensitivity to external states implies the flow and exchange of information. Information is however not like energy, which is covered by the energy equations of physics and the corresponding enthalpy equations of chemistry. Rather, information is more like a *switch*, turning processes off and on, hence being representable typically by 0s and 1s; or like a gate that has continuous positions between open and shut.

The new concept of information was constructed inside and outside biology. Critical advances were made by logicians, mathematicians and electrical engineers in the 1940s as part of war efforts to break codes and to secure codes. Here is Andrew Hodges on this point, referring to Turing's work in Bletchley and Shannon's in Bell Labs in the early 1940s [4] (p. 317):

> Rapidly developing, and not only in Bletchley and Washington, was a new kind of machinery, a new kind of science, in which it was not the physics and chemistry that mattered, but the logical structure of information, communication, and control.

This sentence summarises the way that current science has taken leave of the old reductionist assumption that only the physics and chemistry of matter. Appropriately, it works across all the sciences, forging links and creating a unity among previously unconnected problem areas. That is to say, the new kind of science works across all the sciences except physics and chemistry, which deal with energy transfer, but even then, it has comprehensible, theorised and technological connections with the physics and chemistry of the processes involved.

The logical rules of information flow—such as 'if A then B'—can take, as first approximation, energy values as initial state variables, for example, electrical potential difference across the mitochondrial membrane, but the consequents are regulatory variables—such as open or close, or open or close more or less. This points to the need to correct the first approximation of the initial state variables: they are not energy values, but information about them. It is the information that triggers the regulatory response. In interacting control mechanisms, the initial states are also regulatory variables—another gate being open or closed, and so on. Implementation of such rules requires suitable materials in a suitable state—it might be difficult to make a switch out of a cup of water for example—but apart from this entirely crucial qualification, material composition is unimportant. Another way of making this point is that the energy transfer involved in information transfer is irrelevant to the information transfer. The flow of information depends on regularities, but these regularities are not determined by the energy equations of physics and chemistry, rather they must rely on other properties of materiality. The concept required at this point is expressed by such terms as *structure, form*, *shape* or *syntax* (to borrow from logic)—that *codes information*. The concept of code, reliant on form or shape, signifies how biology breaks away from physics. Code is fallible, liable to error, and it has an arbitrary quality: the same information can be carried by different forms. Code is a kind of mechanism: it makes things happen in the receiving system, and what it makes happen depends on the state of the emitting system.

In short, for life to arise and persist requires much organising and control of the physics and chemistry, and this organising and control relies on information. Here is the oncologist Siddhartha Mukherjee in his book *The Gene: An Intimate History* referring to similar points [5] (p. 409):

> The universe seeks equilibriums; it prefers to disperse energy, disrupt organisation, and maximise chaos. Life is designed to combat these forces. We slow down reactions, concentrate matter, and organise chemicals into compartments…

Mukherjee goes on to emphasise the importance of the *circular flow of biological information*: Genes *encode* RNAs, *to build* Proteins, to *form/ regulate* Organisms, *that sense* Environments, *that influence* Proteins, RNA (and DNA), that regulate Genes….—commenting that it is 'perhaps one of the few organising principles in biology, the closest thing that we might have to biological law' [5] (p. 410).

To sum up, current biological models include both biochemistry, subject to physico-chemical energy equations, *plus* models of information-based regulatory control mechanisms. Here is an illustration of such mechanisms, from a paper titled 'Signaling in Control of Cell Growth and Metabolism' [6].

> In multicellular organisms, cell growth and proliferation are normally not cell autonomous. Receptor-mediated signal transduction, initiated by extracellular growth factors, promotes entry into the cell cycle and reprograms cellular metabolism to fulfil the biosynthetic needs of cell growth and division […] However, despite having become highly dependent on instruction from extracellular growth factors, mammalian cells have retained the ability to sense their internal metabolic reserves and adjust their growth and biosynthetic activities accordingly. Much of this feedback control occurs at the level of posttranslational modifications of signal transduction proteins by key cellular metabolites. Moreover, intracellular metabolites can also regulate chromatin accessibility to control gene expression…

This quotation illustrates, as would so many others, the fundamental and dominant importance of regulatory control processes in current biological/biomedical science.

As already implied, the appearance of regulatory control processes in biology, in addition to the energy-related equations of physics and chemistry, has major implications for the unity of science, paving the way for interacting linkages between the biological, the psychological and the social. This is because elaborations of these processes are found throughout these domains. As illustration, consider this passage from Lane, proposing a reason why mitochondria retain their own local genes [3] (p. 187):

> The mitochondrial genes must be right there on site, next to the bioenergetic membranes they serve. I'm told that the political term is 'bronze control'… In a war, gold control is the central government, which shapes long-term strategy; silver control is the army command, who planned the distribution of manpower or weaponry used; but a war is won or lost on the ground, under the command of bronze control, the brave men or women who actually engage enemy, take the tactical decisions, who inspire their troops, and who are remembered in history as great soldiers. Mitochondrial genes are bronze control, decision-makers on the ground…

This illustrates how new explanatory concepts now fundamental to biology, apply also to psychological and social processes. Or it can be put the other way round: when biophysicists want to explain their theoretical models, they help themselves to processes and principles familiar in psychosocial phenomena. The idea of theory reduction to basic science has disappeared.

Error Is Fundamental to Biology

Control of energetic, metabolic processes is what holds back entropy increase, keeping biological organisms alive and functioning, as opposed to back to dust. The next point to emphasise is that control processes, dependent on information transfer, can go wrong, unlike energy transfers, which can't. Here is Lane explaining further the need for local genetic control, 'decision-making', in energy production in the mitochondria [3] (p. 187):

> Why are such decisions necessary? [...] We discussed the sheer power of the proton-motive force. The mitochondrial membrane has an electrical potential of about 150–200 millivolts. As the membrane is just 5 nanometres thick, [...] this translates into a field strength of 30 million volts per metre, equal to a bolt of lightning. Woe betide you if you lose control over such an electrical charge!

Loss of control leads to poor outcomes [3] (pp. 187–188):

> The penalty is not simply a loss of ATP synthesis, although that alone may well be serious. Failure to transfer electrons properly down the respiratory chains to oxygen (or other electron receptors) can result in a kind of electrical short-circuiting, in which electrons escape to react directly with oxygen or nitrogen, to form reactive 'free radicals'. The combination of falling ATP levels, depolarisation of the bioenergetic membranes and release of free radicals is the classic trigger for 'programmed cell death'... In essence, mitochondrial genes can respond to local changes in conditions, modulating the membrane potential within modest bounds before changes become catastrophic.

The general conceptual point at issue here is that regulation and control mechanisms keep things going *right rather than wrong*. Such normativity is not present in the energy equations of physics and chemistry, which always apply and never fail. It arises in biology for the first time, marking a fundamental departure of biology from physical and chemical processes alone. The normativity is implied in all of the key systems theoretic concepts such as *regulation*, *control* and *information*. It derives from the point that biological systems function towards ends, and function well and badly accordingly as they do or do not attain them. In the present illustration the point is that if electrical charge in the cell membrane is not properly regulated, the cell dies.

Normativity applies at the basic level of genetic replication, as for example in 'transcription error' in molecular genetics—or 'mutation' as used in evolutionary biology. The concept of mutation is critical in evolutionary biology, crucial to explaining how diversity arises—the condition for natural selection processes to operate. Genes are the vehicles of information passed from one generation to the next, including the required building instructions; they normally run true, creating like for like, but to explain diversity they have to be able to mutate, to make a mistake in the replication. It was a hard question what shape of thing could have these and this combination of functional qualities—the answer turning out to be the double helix. Watson and Crick's [7] double-helix structure could replicate itself (by a several stage process), securing continuity, and it could also mutate, delivering a copy with a changed order of bases. This variation leads to production of different proteins that could (might or might not) affect the phenotype interacting with the environment, which difference could (might or might not) differentially affect survival and propagation. But this variation at the phenotypic level is possible because variation is possible at the molecular level, because various nucleotide sequences are possible, all consistent with complex molecular thermodynamic equilibrium. The emergence of biological diversity depends on the kind of error that genes are capable of.

As implicit above, normativity also applies at the level of the whole organism in interaction with the environment: interaction is *adaptive* insofar as it promotes continuity and functioning and is otherwise *maladaptive*. Evolution depends on these two kinds of normativity—genetic mutation and adaptation. These kinds of normativity are biologically fundamental, based on scope for error. Cell respiration is disrupted if sufficient oxygen fails to be delivered; defence mechanisms in a cell can mistake a virus for a metabolite or other signalling molecule; or elements detected in viral particles cause the human immune system to attack a tissue or cell which would normally be treated as self and not subject to immune attack, with resultant inflammatory response and immune inflicted damage, up to and including cell death. Error arises in many ways, one of which, just referred to, is that the competition can deceive by mimicking, from viruses on upwards. Life and diversity are closely linked, one upshot being that the same or diverse life forms typically end up in competition for finite energy resources. The competition exploits the possibility of error in information transfer that is fundamental to life forms. All these goings on do not matter at all to the energy equations of physics and chemistry—everything conforms to them—but some do matter to the biology, hence there is pervasive use for normative contrasts: 'functions well/badly' 'right'/'wrong', 'same'/'error', life/death, health/disease.

Life Forms: Diversity Amidst the Physics

Living systems exploit slack—they find options within—physical laws. At the basic level of genes there are diverse complex molecules, all thermodynamically stable, consistent with physical, quantum-mechanical energy equations, but which are interestingly different, because they may have very different consequences for the organism, positive or negative. This much transforms the explanatory framework, but also the ontology, which includes not only physical material, but shapes or forms such as double helixes, with their novel causal properties of regulatory control, programming and replication.

The possibility of proliferation of forms and causal potentials within the constraints of physical, quantum-mechanical energy equations is well illustrated in the genetic code and genetic replication, but it has wide application. It can be seen already in chemistry, in the diversity of the elements, in their diverse structures, resulting in variety in physical properties (such as melting and boiling points), and in chemical combinatorial properties, all of which are consistent with energy equations. All of the chemical elements, and the great diversity of their combinations, including the complex molecules in biological systems, all conform to the equations—but the critical point is that the equations permit chemical diversity and complexity including those in biological processes.

Diversity arises from increasing complexity, successions of combinations of parts into greater wholes. The parts essentially interact with one another—otherwise they would not make a whole thing, but would remain isolated separate things. The wholes become parts of other wholes—and so on. This can be seen in physics, where subatomic particles interactively form into atoms, and in chemistry, where atoms compound into molecules. In biology, all the physics and chemistry continue to apply, but new phenomena appear: regulation of physico-chemical processes by coded information—and with that, especially the possibility of error. Concepts of error gain traction in relation to wider systems and functional ends of those systems—ultimately responsible for natural biological systems being able—in local areas, temporarily—to avoid the general increase of entropy, to increase energy differences, to make more order out of less order.

The increasingly larger and more complex *shapes*, *structures* or *forms*, have distinctive new causal properties. *Form* here is dynamical, a matter of what the molecule, cell or membrane can do and does. For example, the fusion effects of intense gravity in collapsing stars make new things from hydrogen, metals such as iron, a new structure with new physical and chemical properties—and among the elements necessary for life. Once life gets going, diversity takes on a whole new meaning: countless new structures, forms, complexity, capacities and operating principles. Biological processes exploit the physics and chemistry from the start, for example the physics of proton gradient across a cell membrane, or energy released according to chemical enthalpy equations in Krebs' cycle. At the complex molecular level, shape (structure) is critical to distinguishing them and determining their interactive properties. As one moves to complex organic and biochemical molecules, shape is increasingly exploited. In cellular biology for example, the function of enzyme catalysts turns on their shape and fit to relevant biochemical agents—as in 'lock and key' models. Biological forms not only conform to physics and chemical energy equations, they manage the energetic processes, with new principles of regulation and information flow. These biological principles operate in the very large spaces permitted by those energy equations, producing new forms on top of the physical elements and chemical combinations that those laws permit. And with the new forms come new operating principles, though what remains at their core are the original components: the need for energy, for preservation, the critical importance of regulation and information flow.

The above issues are linked to the concept of 'emergence' which has a long history in the philosophy of biology and psychology, and systems theory generally. For review of the topic, see e.g. [8]. There are detailed treatments in recent philosophy of biology (e.g. [9, 10]).

The new biology, employing causal principles that turn on shape or form in relation to systemic ends, marks a radical departure from physicalism that has its roots in the seventeenth-century mechanisation of the world picture. These developments also, as is well known, point backwards to the science and philosophy that preceded the development of seventeenth-century science, specifically to Aristotle. Aristotle had a broad vision of causation, comprising 4 kinds: *material*, *efficient*, *formal* and *final*, arguing that formal and final causes were likely to be especially relevant to biological processes (see, e.g., Andrea Falcon's critical review [11]). The new seventeenth mechanics, however, required—in these terms—only the first two, while the second two dropped out of the science as redundant. When biological sciences developed in the nineteenth century, research programmes emulated the natural sciences, discovering the chemistry within biological processes. However, reducing the phenomena to chemistry was not such a clear option for other parts of biology, especially study of the formation of whole organisms and whole species: *embryology* and *evolutionary biology*. These have always seemed to require concepts different from those in the natural sciences, more akin to Aristotle's formal and final causes.

It was always *final* or *teleological* explanation that was the most problematic for natural science. It seems to imply that the *ends* must in some way be *already present at the start*, and it has been assumed—notwithstanding Aristotle's original disavowal [11]—that this could only be so if the ends are in some way 'preconceived' by some purposive intelligence/designer. It is probably true that teleological explanation of a change supposes that the end-conditions must somehow be present at the beginning, and it is also true that genes do not in any way 'have in mind' the proteins they produce. It is however exactly at this point that the information-processing paradigm does its conceptual work, because the genes *encode (code for)* the proteins they produce. In this sense—the sense of *encoding*—the ends are already present at the start—and in this sense the information-processing model envisages—something like—teleological explanation. A typical explanation in the information-processing paradigm is that particular genes code for particular proteins. Needless to say much hangs on what 'code for' means. But what it does not mean is that some protein-like shape already exists in the genes, obviously still less that the genetic material has a mental image of the proteins to be produced. Rather, 'code for' means: in normal circumstances, in the normal cellular environment, in a complex series of interlocking steps, such-and-such DNA sequence produces such-and-such protein. The coding concept secures the idea that the 'ends' are already present—in some sense—and are instrumental in production (under normal circumstances) of the end result. This dynamic, production sense of 'encoded information' is more explicitly captured by terms like 'programme' or 'instructions', with clearer implication of direction to an end, and connotes more clearly that the production process follows rules (if… then…)

that are not inviolable physico-chemical laws but violable metabolic regularities.

In summary, the information-processing paradigm in biology secures the fundamental point that the functional end of a system—the result it tends in normal circumstances to produce—is in a defined sense already present in the system prior to production, as instructions and a mechanism for the production. These kinds of principles of causal explanation involving forms and ends were anticipated by Aristotle, as was the insight that they are likely to apply particularly in biology.

The concept of genetic coding recreates a refined, scientific version of the idea that the ends are—as programming instructions—present at the start. No such idea, however, is implied by Darwin's theory: on the contrary, evolution as envisaged by Darwin does not admit of a teleological type of explanation in any sense, but rather provides a quite different alternative in terms of random genetic mutation, adaptation and natural selection. Once natural (as opposed to human made) functional systems come into being, they admit of teleological explanation, expressed in the idea that states of biological systems encode—instructions for—production processes. Genes coding for embryonic development is a fundamental example. But no analogue of the information-processing paradigm applies to evolution as a whole; the *teleologic* applies only to systems with design—forms suited to securing particular ends—that result from the evolutionary process, not to the evolutionary process itself.

2.2 The Limitations of Physicalism

Preamble and the Argument in Brief Lay Terms

This is the most explicitly philosophical section of the book because it addresses positions in the contemporary analytic philosophy literature where physicalism holds an important place. The whole section may be less accessible and of less interest to the reader without background knowledge of philosophy, but we include it here because physicalism is of fundamental importance to the conceptualisation of the sciences and how they relate to one another, in turn therefore of fundamental importance to understanding the conceptual foundations of the biopsychosocial model. The importance of physicalism in Engel's original formulation of the biomedical model, some historical expressions of physicalism, and the recognition by current commentators of the need for distinctive biopsychosocial causal interactions—were reviewed as context for the general biopsychosocial model at the beginning of Sect. 1.3.

Physicalism in its clearest, strong version holds that everything that there is and all causation is physical, or, alternatively expressed: everything is physical, covered by physical laws. This doctrine exerts massive downwards reductionist pressure on all other sciences: their ontology and their causal principles ultimately have to be physical, or else illusionary. Chemistry passes under the bar, much of biology is physics and chemistry, psychology is problematic, and social science even more so. All are basically bad news for any biopsychosocial model. Or the other way round, a viable biopsychosocial model is bad news for physicalism.

The key step in the shift away from physicalism and physicalist reductionism occurs in current biology and has been examined in the previous section. In brief, current biology since the mid-twentieth century envisages not only physical and chemical energetic processes but also regulatory control of those processes. Crucially: regulatory control mechanisms never contravene the energy equations of physics and chemistry (because nothing ever does), but it is a type of causation. Regulatory control mechanisms are typically dynamical forms, the causal properties of which turn on shape as opposed to material constituent parts. This is clear in the cosmic prize-winning case of the complex molecular DNA double helix, and evident in the supporting cast of, for example, enzymes working like keys in locks. From here, once dynamical life forms with regulatory control functions take off from the physics and chemistry of the matter, from compliance with energy equations alone, they become ever more complex and diverse in evolution, to include eventually psychological and social phenomena. There are certainly reasons to distinguish regulatory control by genes and enzymes from regulatory control by nervous systems, from regulatory control by social rules and regulations, but the key thing from a philosophical point of view is that they can all be conceptualised under this very general heading, they can causally interact, and especially, they are not tied down by, though always compliant with, the energy equations of physics and chemistry. In short, the ontology and causal theory of current biology can envisage psychological and social processes, making the biopsychosocial model viable.

This, in brief, is the argument we propose to work around physicalism. The rest of the section is more philosophically technical and detailed.

Physicalism

Physicalism and related reductionism have been extensively discussed in contemporary analytic philosophy during the past few decades. It would be fair to say that they are mainstream views, but also challenged, defended and modified. While the challenges are substantial, it would be fair to say, nevertheless, that physicalism has no serious competitors, no viable, large scale alternatives. Such alternatives as are envisaged in this mainstream literature, the philosophies to which physicalism is opposed—dualism and vitalism—are historical and long discredited in the science. We suggest that contemporary alternatives are to be found in current biological theory, key features of which, it will be argued in subsequent chapters, carry into psychology and behavioural science.

In broad terms, physicalism is the view that everything is physical and there is nothing else besides. This ontology most obviously would comprise a view as to causation and causal laws, namely, that all causation and all causal laws are physical, or another way of putting this: 'physics explains everything'. This would seem to follow clearly enough: since there are only physical events, there are only physical events to explain, so the only explanations are physical. Or again: physical things have physical causal powers, and therefore, since there are only physical things, there are only physical causal powers. The matters of ontology and causation should probably be tied together in a tight knot. *If* there seemed to be only physical things, and *if* we had only physical causal explanations, then the physicalist metaphysics would stay as simple as this. The broad problem for physicalism is just that these two conditions have never held. It has never seemed like there were only physical things, and never that we explained everything by physics. The ontological problem was and remains easily enough disposed of by saying: it may seem that there are many kinds of non-physical things—animation, perceptions—but these are only appearances, and they are really physical things, or just appearances, and not real after all. Similar moves can be made about apparent causes and effects, especially mind over body: the causation is illusory, or really physical.

The one place at which this imperious dogmatising falters is where apparently non-physical entities and causal processes are invoked by empirical sciences, finding associations and following methods for determination of causes articulated by Mill. Just as the real backing for the mechanisation of the world picture and the beginnings of physicalism was success of the science, mechanics, it can only be undermined by more else of the same, i.e. more but different successful science. These new sciences were established in the nineteenth century with advances through the twentieth: chemistry, biology, psychology, social sciences—with all their large and small sub-fields.

As these new sciences developed, physicalism becomes entangled with *reductionism*: the assumption that, and the project of trying to show that, these new sciences can be reduced to physics; meaning, that their ontology and causal principles can or could ultimately be eliminated in favour of the physical. Such strong reduction—in an ideal physicalist world, elimination—known as, for example, semantic- or theory- reduction, has not however fared well. It does well in chemistry, in parts of physiology, struggles seriously in psychology, and is hopeless in social science. As noted in Sect. 1.3, under the heading "Theorising Biopsychosocial Interactions—Not Parallel Worlds", by around the 1970s, something of a halt was called, with acknowledgement that the sciences apart from physics–chemistry, over and above them, what Fodor called the 'Special Sciences', could not be reduced/eliminated, and there were, after all, causal concepts and principles, over and above those of physics [12–14]

That might have spelt the end of physicalism, except for the option, unattractive but needs must, of disconnecting ontology from causation and causal explanation. Physicalism could be retained as a view of what stuff there is—only physical—while acknowledging that, where theory or semantic reductionism fails, there are constructs of non-physical entities, processes and causes in the sciences above physics–chemistry. This depleted version of physicalism as an ontological doctrine only—not about causes—has a corresponding weaker reductionist doctrine, called *ontological*, or *metaphysical*, without commitment to *epistemological* or *explanatory reduction*, and the combination is sometimes called 'non-reductive physicalism' [see, e.g., 15]. Insofar as this weaker form of Physicalism is an ontological claim only, involving no claims about causal explanations, it probably has given up on being much or anything to do with the sciences, and becomes a purely 'metaphysical' doctrine.

As suggested above, however, the move of separating off ontology from causation is very awkward, requiring as it does a conception of things (entities, properties or processes) somehow independent of what they do, independent of their causal powers and interactions. The awkwardness shows up in various related ways. Consider mental states, the traditional anomaly for physicalism: if—in the ontological version of physicalism—they are allowed to be causal, connected by psychological principles not physical laws, what account can be given of their ontological status—given that the assumption that the only ontology is physical?

The basic problem is not ontological however—we can say what we like about what there is, if this makes no commitment to causal properties—rather, the basic problem involves theorising causation. While non-reductive physicalism seeks to acknowledge non-physical causes, it still retains physical causal laws, implicitly including a massive theory of causation, but since these physical laws cover all physical processes, and since these are the only events that there are, then the difficult question arises: where is there any room for causation by anything else, by mental events for example (whatever may be their curious ontological status)? The ontological issues in contemporary physicalism are often theorised in terms of 'supervenience' and the conundrum in the theory of causation as to how there can be mental causes as well as physical causes is sometimes called the 'dual causation' or 'causal overdetermination' problem (see, e.g., [16, 17]).

The many types of physicalist 'reductionism' that have had to be invoked in this philosophical literature, outlined above, indicate just how much it has struggled to survive in the current scientific climate. The depleted version left at the end is ontological only, seeking to subtract commitments on causality, although actually retaining the assumption that physical causation covered by physical laws is the only kind. It is this assumed 'completeness of physics' that actually delivers the core, best argument for physicalism, and we consider it next.

Regulatory Mechanisms Do Not Affect Energy Equations

There is a core argument for physicalism based on the so-called causal completeness of physical. This argument is for a strong form of physicalism in that sense that it would prohibit the idea of any non-physical cause making a difference to energy and energy exchanges of physical material. Here is the philosopher David Papineau presenting the argument, in several stages corresponding to historical developments in the science [18] (p. 9):

> In the middle of the nineteenth century the conservation of kinetic plus potential energy came to be accepted as a basic principle of physics… In itself this does not did rule out fundamental mental or vital forces… but … does imply that any such special forces must be governed by strict deterministic laws to ensure they never led to energy increases.
>
> During the course of the twentieth century received scientific opinion became even more restrictive about possible causes of physical effects, and came to reject *sui generis* mental or vital causes, even of a law governed and predictable kind. Detailed physiological research, especially into nerve cells, gave no indication of any physical effects that cannot be explained in terms of basic physical forces that also occur outside living bodies. By the middle of the twentieth century, belief in sui generis mental or vital forces had become a minority view. This led to the widespread acceptance of the doctrine now known as the "causal closure" or the "causal completeness of the physical", according to which all physical effects have fully physical causes.

This is a powerful argument in favour of physicalism. Tracking the science, it successfully excludes non-physical forces capable of making energy differences. Physicalism wins if the opposing team is 'spooky' energy-exchanging forces, as in dualism and vitalism.

Current biology and biomedicine, however, go off at a tangent to this problematic. As outlined in the preceding section, the new life sciences envisage distinctive forms, structures and information-based regulatory control mechanisms—in addition to energy exchanges and conservation covered by the equations of physics. However, and of course, this departure from physics respects the physical energy equations. In short, there are distinctive biological structures and causes—regulatory mechanisms—but they don't interfere with the physics; they exploit the physics, rely on it, manage it—but they don't change it.

Consider the analogy of a chemical industrial plant running, for example, the Haber process for production of ammonia from hydrogen and nitrogen. The model of the process certainly includes the core chemical reactions and the associated enthalpy (energy) equations. However, for the chemical reaction to run at all, to run forwards and not too much backwards, the hydrogen and nitrogen have to be present in quantities in an appropriate range, at temperature and pressure high enough, though not too high for the containers, aided by the presence of catalysts. The model of all this includes regulatory control mechanisms for delivery and removal of materials, temperature and pressure control, etc. Several points can be noted:

> First, the regulatory control mechanisms never affect energy exchange equations and never flout the principle of conservation of energy. They obviously don't because nothing does—but in any case they don't.
>
> Second, the chemical reactions can occur outside the factory. Equally the basic energy exchange physico-chemical reactions in, for example, biological cells could occur outside of cells.
>
> Third, as a qualification, in both cases, they only occur—inside or outside the factory—if the necessary reactants come together in a particular sequence, particular amounts, at particular temperatures, etc. Bringing this about—in the chemical industrial factory, as in the biological cell—requires substantial organisational and control mechanisms.

The physical/chemical energy equations cover some aspects of the Haber process: how much energy is absorbed or produced, etc. The principles of regulatory control model other aspects, answering questions such as: 'how is the rate of reaction kept within a range, so as not to run too fast or too hot?', 'Why does this gate shut at this time, cutting off the supply of hydrogen?' There will be a physical process that shuts the gate, but, if the gate shutting is part of a regulatory mechanism (is indeed a 'gate shutting'), it will involve a physical process that can 'go wrong'. For example, the gate has a particular shape, and the process that shuts it may be the arrival of an object which fits it like a key; the key turning in the lock is a physical process, and it does not violate any physical equations, because nothing does, but the process is also a regulatory one, signified by the fact that it can go wrong, because for example the key has a fault in it, or because there are competitor saboteurs at work with fake keys. Models of regulatory control mechanisms are distinct from physico-chemical equations covering energy exchanges; they are a different kind of causal-explanatory framework, suited to different processes, answering different sorts of question.

As a corollary, there is no problem of 'dual causation' or 'causal over-determination'. In the present context the problem would be: how can a regulatory mechanism cause anything when all the causing is already accomplished by physical events covered by physical laws? But the problem doesn't arise because regulatory mechanisms do not concern energy exchanges covered by physical laws. Nowhere in these models (in chemical engineering or biology) is the same process being causally explained twice.

The benefits of models of causation by regulatory control extend to promoting research questions, supporting predictions, enabling control, diagnosis of dysfunctions and fixing things. For example, if the model of regulatory control of a chemical factory includes that a particular gate opens or closes depending on the rate of reaction relative to parameters of temperature and pressure, the model can be used to predict when the gate will open or close. The model also prompts a research programme to investigate the mechanisms by which the gate is sensitive within certain ranges to the rate of reaction, temperature and pressure. If the plant blows up, we want to know why. Generally, the model guides understanding of dysfunction or breakdown. If, for example, the reaction is running too hot, becoming inefficient or raising risk of meltdown—the model tells us that one cause might be malfunctioning of a gate, for example, the hinges are rusted, or the thermostatic devices regulating its function are malfunctioning. We can also use the model to intervene, for example, in the case of dysfunction one might fix the rust or the regulatory feedback mechanism. Use of such models is obvious enough in chemical engineering and the analogues pervade physiology and biomedicine.

It may be objected: 'but factories have designs that promote functional ends, but they are human built—not natural systems'. But this is a pre-Darwinian thought. Natural systems, biological ones, have this kind of design—regulatory control mechanisms—resulting from random mutation and natural selection.

Causation by regulatory control has distinctive properties, among the most curious of which is causation by events that don't happen! This phenomenon has been theorised in current philosophy of causation and is taken up below. First we give reasons why the weakest form of physicalism, really limited to an ontological claim only, without any presumption about causation, is unattractive.

Weaker—Ontological Only—Physicalism Is Problematic

In their Stanford Encyclopedia entry on Supervenience, Brian McLaughlin and Karen Bennett, in the section titled 'Coincident Entities and the "Grounding Problem"', consider the classic example of a lump of clay (Lumpl) later fashioned into a statue (Goliath), which have different modal properties—such as that the one survives being squashed into a ball while the other does not—which seems to entail they are different things [19] (p. 51), continuing:

> The main objection to the view that Goliath and Lumpl are distinct is what can be called 'the grounding problem'. How can Lumpl and Goliath differ in their modal properties, given that they are alike in every other way? What grounds their difference in persistence conditions? In virtue of what do they have the persistence conditions they do?

The obvious way in which the lump of clay and the statue are the same is that they are made of the same material. The obvious way they differ is in shape or form. According to the view we have argued for in this chapter, shape or form, over and above material composition, can be of critical importance in determining causal properties. This is less evident in the classic lump of clay/statue example, because statues do not have standout causal powers over and above those due to their material composition. However, if we shift the example to the DNA double-helix dynamical form, which, in its normal operating environment, has amazing causal properties such as replication and coding for protein production. These properties could be reasonably called 'emergent' in the sense that they are not evident in the formless, unorganised higher entropic sum of its elements.

This line of thought implies that the very weak form of physicalism as an ontological claim only, about 'metaphysical grounding', is bound to be deficient. Shamik Dasgupta writes [20] (p. 557):

> It has been suggested that many philosophical theses—physicalism, nominalism, normative naturalism, and so on—should be understood in terms of ground… What is physicalism? Not just physicalism about the mind, but physicalism period. What kind of a thesis is it? We know what the rough picture is: at some basic level the world is constituted wholly out of physical stuff, and everything else—football matches, string quartets, consciousness, values, numbers—somehow 'arises out of' that physical stuff. Or, to use other locutions, everything else is "fixed by" or 'determined by' or 'is nothing over and above' that physical stuff. Or, as the metaphor goes, all God had to do when making the world was make the physical stuff, and then her job was done.

The last sentence seems to imply that nothing interesting, or nothing at all, has happened since the fraction of second after the Big Bang—or, staying with its metaphor, the sentence neglects what God made on all the other days. The formations and phases of stars, formation of elements, metals, complex molecules, conditions for life on at least one planet, the whole evolutionary process of organisms and of mammals and primates—have what status according to this metaphysical grounding thesis? Presumably the grounding thesis allows that such things exist, now or past, but limits itself to a claim about what these things are constituted out of, and this in a highly reductive sense, which recognises only what is common between hydrogen and iron for example, and not their differences including their different combinatorial and causal properties; or again which admits only what is common between metallic iron and biological tissue, not their differences, including their different causal properties, such as that metallic iron contains no regulatory mechanisms, but biological tissue does. However, Dasgupta supposes that this minimalist ontology can have explanatory value, indeed—curiously—'full' explanatory value [20] (p. 558):

> To say that some facts ground another is just to say that the former explain the latter, in a particular sense of 'explain'. When I say that some facts ground another, I mean that the former fully explain the latter.

'Fully explain' is too strong however, if we wish to explain not only the material similarity between hydrogen, iron and biological cells but also the differences in their causal properties. It can be said that specifying what material something is made of explains it to some extent—though probably only because its causal properties are being assumed, for example mechanical properties of physical matter; but there are so many other things and causal properties to explain, such as chemical combinatorial possibilities and properties that turn on structure, or systemic functioning that turns on achieving or maintaining end states. In short, there is need for a principled variety of kinds of explanation, of which Aristotle's typology of causes, briefly reviewed at the end of the preceding section, is the original. In those terms, physicalism can be regarded as a weak ontological claim only, specifying the material cause of everything as physical. In these terms there are however in addition efficient causes, an approximate example being the operation of mechanical forces, and formal and final causes (dynamical forms that tend to an end-state) that have a particular explanatory role to play in modelling biological systems.

Causation by Events That Don't Happen

Recent novel philosophical analyses of causation have drawn attention to the curious fact that some causal pathways involve events that do not happen! This is a very clear sign of causation that does not involve energy transfer.

Jonathan Schaffer begins his paper titled 'Causation by Disconnection' like this [21] (p. 285):

> It is widely believed that causation requires a *connection* from cause to effect, such as an energy flow. But there are many ways to wire a causal mechanism. One way is to have the cause connect to the effect, but another is to have the cause disconnect what was blocking the effect.

Using the example of a bomb detonation mechanism, Schaffer points out that it can be wired in various ways, including: pressing the button generates an electrical current which connects to the bomb and makes it explode, or pressing the button disconnects an electrical current that was inhibiting an independent source from triggering the explosion. Schaffer notes the similarities between this latter case of causation by disconnection and other recent approaches to causation, such as Ned Hall's on causation by 'double prevention', involving absence of events or 'negative' causation [22, 23]. In short, this recent philosophical work identifies a kind of causal connection—variously identified as 'disconnection', 'negative', 'double prevention'—that is not a matter of energy flow.

The important point for our present purpose is that the examples of this other kind of causal connection all involve *functional mechanisms*, whether artefacts, or natural, biological systems. Schaffer uses detonator wiring diagrams, but the footnote explaining the diagram conventions refer to neuronal firing or not-firing, stimulatory and inhibitory connections [21] (p. 286n). In other words, we are dealing here with *biological causation*. James Woodward in his *Making Things Happen* notes that there are many scientific examples of causation by double prevention, particularly in biology, giving as illustration Jacob and Monod's *lac operon* model for *Escherichia coli*, noting that biologists describe this as a case of 'negative control' [24] (pp. 225–226). This clearly illustrates that causation by double prevention is situated within the explanatory paradigm of regulatory control so far outlined.

The idea of causal pathways that involve absences of events is probably tied inextricably to the systems theoretic concepts of functioning towards ends and contributions of part functioning to whole functioning. In this context whole functioning will depend on whether inputs are or are not received from another part, and both cases are of interest. So, for example, closing of a gate and the consequent cessation of delivery of a chemical into a chemical reaction container, is as interesting as the gate being open—otherwise there would be no point in using the term 'gate'. Distinctions like open/closed, happens/doesn't happen are integral to the normativity of regulatory control, and they have no analogue in physico-chemical laws/equations covering energy exchanges.

The critical point is that all these curious kinds of explanations posited in recent philosophical work on causation—'disconnection', 'negative', 'double prevention'—are to be distinguished from causal connections that rely on energy transformation and conservation. The standard philosophical view about causation has been to emphasise this latter kind of causal connection. Schaffer [21] (p. 286) attributes this standard view widely, to Wesley Salmon, Phil Dowe, Peter Menzies and David Armstrong. In a strong form, the proposal is to limit causal processes as those that transmit conserved quantities—the clearest example of which is energy in physics. The new work in philosophy of causation is consistent with the approach we have taken in this chapter, which distinguishes regulatory control from energy transformations and conservation covered by physical equations.

Philosophy of Biology Notes

Recent philosophy of biology has focussed on systems theoretic concepts and principles, such as (*dynamical*) *systems/mechanisms*, *part/whole relationships and complexity*. Books include William Bechtel and Robert C. Richardson's *Discovering Complexity: Decomposition and Localization as Strategies in Scientific Research* [10]; Sandra D. Mitchell's *Biological Complexity and Integrative Pluralism* [25]; and William C. Wimsatt's *Re-engineering Philosophy for Limited Beings* [9]. This is a very rich literature dealing with many topics in philosophy of biology, including those few covered here, in much more detail, and with many examples.

The different focus here is the philosophy of biology as it defines key conceptual features of the first component of the biopsychosocial, especially to bring out that the key conceptual features of current biology open up the way to a coherent view of biopsychosocial ontology and causation appropriate for the biopsychosocial model of health and disease. For this purpose we have emphasised the relation of biology to physics–chemistry and especially the fundamental role of information as well as energy, the theory started by Erwin Schrödinger, picked up by Ludwig von Bertalanffy, and used in contemporary biophysics and genetics by for example Nick Lane and Siddhartha Mukherjee. Generally this line of thought has not been the focus in philosophy of biology. Moreover, there are some signs of antipathy towards it in the mainstream philosophical literature, directed against the core notion of *information*, as considered next.

Biological Information Is Semantic (Capable of Error)

We noted at some length in Sect. 2.1, under the heading "Error Is Fundamental to Biology", that normativity, including the possibility of error, is fundamental to biological regulatory control mechanisms. Normativity is however entirely anomalous for physicalism. Physicalism envisages only the few physical qualities, related to mass, momentum, energy—and it especially doesn't envisage any of the family that includes (*semantic*) *information* or *intentionality*, characterises by *aboutness* or *directness*, and the *possibility of error*. Here for example is Jerry Fodor [26] (p. 97):

> The deepest motivation for intentional irrealism derives… from a certain ontological intuition: that there is no place for intentional categories in a physicalist view of the world; that the intentional can't be naturalised.

This ontological intuition is correct: biological information, bound up with regulation and the possibility of error, has no place in the physicalist view of the world, assuming this envisages only energy exchanges and the physical laws/equations that govern them. Hence there is enormous pressure from physicalism to disqualify or down-grade the information-processing paradigm in biology, specifically to deny the possibility of error. This is actually quite difficult to do since subtract information-processing concepts, always involving normativity, from contemporary biology textbooks and there is practically nothing left.

The disqualification move is especially unattractive in the case of genes and genetic information. This suggests a compromise of limiting error-prone information to genes. Here for example is Paul Griffiths [27] (p. 295):

> There is a genetic code by which the sequence of DNA bases in the coding regions of a gene corresponds to the sequence of amino acids in the primary structure of one or more proteins… The rest of 'information talk' in biology is no more than a picturesque way to talk about correlation and causation.

Such a concession is philosophically pointless however; it only takes a single exception—though in this case by the way a massive one (genetics/life)—to disprove the metaphysical claim that there is no error-prone information in nature.

Another possibility is to envisage semantic information processing in the mind–brain but not elsewhere in biology, except perhaps, again, in genes. William Bechtel [28] for example highlights the concept of information in the stronger semantic sense in modelling the mind/brain. In a section entitled *Mental Mechanisms: Mechanisms That Process Information*, Bechtel argues that biological phenomena such as cellular respiration 'can be adequately characterised as involving physical transformations of material substances' [28] (p. 22), while 'mental mechanisms are ones that can be investigated taking a physical stance (examining neural structures and their operations) but also, distinctively and crucially, taking an information processing stance' [28] (p. 23). In this discussion, Bechtel qualifies the proposal that sub-mental/neuronal biology has no information processing, making an exception, like Griffiths as quoted above, of genetics [28] (p. 22n).

However, the information-processing and with it the possibility of error in genes, and also in the brain, are not biological exceptional cases, but are rather the rule. The same applies all over the body—for example, to the endocrine system's management of many internal functions, described for example here [29]:

> The endocrine system is a network of glands that secrete chemicals called hormones to help your body function properly. Hormones are chemical signals that coordinate a range of bodily functions. The endocrine system works to regulate certain internal processes… and systems [such as]

growth and development, homeostasis (the internal balance of body systems), metabolism (body energy levels), reproduction, response to stimuli (stress and/or injury).

And—evident in the endocrine disorders—it can all go wrong.

2.3 Current Biomedicine Is Conducive to the Biopsychosocial Model

Consider again Engel's characterisation of the Biomedical Model [30] (p. 130):

> The biomedical model embraces both reductionism, the philosophic view that complex phenomena are ultimately derived from a single primary principle, and mind-body dualism, the doctrine that separates the mental from the somatic. Hence the reductionist primary principle is physicalistic; that is, it assumes that the language of chemistry and physics will ultimately suffice to explain biological phenomena.

Engel uses the term 'reductionism' in this passage in two senses: the first is commitment to there being a single primary principle explaining complex phenomena, specifically a biological principle; the second has to do with the reduction of biology to physics and chemistry. The line of thought in this chapter counts against the complete reduction of biology to physics and chemistry, though retains partial reduction. Much biology relies on the energy exchanges determined by quantum mechanical and chemical combinatorial enthalpy equations. However, these energy exchanges have to be controlled, as do all other biological processes, by regulatory mechanisms involving information transfer. Biology and biomedicine in the last half-century have developed as an exquisite combination of these two kinds of science.

Interestingly, Engel recognised the fundamental role of the new information science in medicine in his 'Foreword' [31] to the book on the subject by Foss and Rothenberg [32]; he acknowledged the shortcomings of the term 'biopsychosocial', which emphasises structural boundaries rather than integration, and welcomed the authors' term 'infomedical'. However while the thinking behind these considerations was sound, this terminology has not caught on, at least not as a replacement for 'biopsychosocial'.

From the systems theory point of view there is no reason at all to quarrel with the partial reduction of biology to physics and chemistry, evidenced in scientific research programmes to determine the biophysics and biochemistry of, for example, cell metabolism or blood oxygen transport. A connected point, nor is there any reason to regard biomedicine as anything other than a scientific medical research programme with a remarkably successful track record. The general direction of biomedical research programmes from the mid-nineteenth century was towards study of internal organs and systems, penetrating beneath, literally inside, the complex presentations of signs and symptoms of disease, and beyond that, deeper inside the bodily organs and systems, to the structure and functioning of cells and the underlying chemistry of molecular processes. Research strategies shifted away from traditional naturalistic observational methods towards laboratory based experimentation, requiring elucidation of experimental methods to determine causation, famously developed in the mid-nineteenth century by Robert Koch in his postulates for use in the new microbiology. Resounding successes in control of infectious diseases and the development of penicillin were followed by many further developments from the mid-twentieth century, in new sciences such as clinical genetics and neuroscience, and new treatment technologies (e.g. [33]).

Biomedical research from the middle of the nineteenth century led the way in understanding the basic physics and chemistry of biological processes, but to this it can be added that since the mid-twentieth century it has also been at the cutting edge of that whole new aspect of biology involving information-based regulatory control mechanisms, the fallibility of which is fundamental to the understanding of disease. In short, and of course, nothing does 'the biological' better than biomedicine. So if the biopsychosocial model wants to include the best concerning the first in its triumvirate, it had better aim to include biomedicine.

On the other hand, in addition, there are also all the other aspects of health, disease and health care that have come to light or prominence over the same period of the last few decades, outlined in Sect. 1.1, which require more than biomedical science. Such as, the epidemiology of social determinants of health, the increasing relative prevalence of non-communicable diseases compared with infectious diseases, raising issues of adjustment and quality of life with chronic health conditions, and broader social changes which have put patient rights and autonomy at the forefront of practice.

This raises the issue of the second type of reductionism that Engel attributed to the biomedical model in the above quotation: reducing complex phenomena to the biological alone. While biology was supposed to reduce to physics and chemistry, and while this supposition had a priori support from physicalism, it would follow fast without much thought that the explanation of diseases, like everything else, would ultimately be in terms of biology = physics and chemistry. Within the confines of physicalism, the possibility of distinctive psychological or social explanatory principles can hardly arise. Conversely, it does arise in a post-physicalist thought space that can envisage psychological and social factors as candidate explanations, as well as biological. In this context, the biomedical assumption that there is a primary biological cause becomes an empirical bet, without a priori, metaphysical/ideological support. The bet is that illnesses have a biological cause—explaining 'most' of the outcome variance. Whether this is true in any given type of illness is a matter for research, and we already know enough to say that it is not true of all illnesses—and not at every stage. This refers to the emerging evidence implicating psychosocial factors reviewed briefly at the beginning of Sect. 1.2.

What is required to comprehend psychosocial reality and causation is a post-physicalist framework that can accommodate more than physics and chemistry. But this is exactly what is opened up by the recent paradigm shift in biology and biomedicine that we have been considering. The main point is that fundamental biological phenomena—form or structure, functioning towards ends, regulatory control and inter-systemic information-transfer—complexify and diversify into what we call the psychological and the social. As noted at the end of the first chapter, under the heading "Developing the General Model", the evolution of life forms ends up with human psychological and social phenomena, but 'ends up with', as currently understood in the science, is not a matter of logic or scientific law, but is entirely contingent—accidental. The original biological function is to maintain biological life, and this preoccupation carries through to the psychological and the social. However, psychological life has conditions in addition to biological life—agency and recognition—and all these matters are managed in forms of social organisation and control. Further, all kinds of biopsychosocial functioning, once we leave the physics and chemistry, are liable to error, vulnerable, illness prone. This expansion into the biopsychosocial conditions of health and disease is the business of the remaining chapters.

A caveat before closing this section: it is clear that there is in the mix a fourth ingredient as well as the biological, psychological and social, namely, 'the environment'. Having our environment identified solely as 'social' is no use at all, not in general, not in any of the life and health sciences. Conceptually from basic genetics and cell biology upwards, it makes no sense to model living processes except in relation to interactions with the environment. This is also the clear context of Schrödinger's linkage between life and the second law of thermodynamics. Certainly it has been clear to the public health physicians that for good health we need food, water, accommodation. The 'biological' and biomedicine imply conditions and interactions with the non-social, physico-chemical environment. However, at the current time 'the environment' demands explicit acknowledgement in any proposed general model of health and disease because of the many urgent environmental challenges we face: threats to global temperature stability, to energy, water and food security, with their impacts on health, and their interactions with social policy. This reflects the increasing importance of geography and environmental sciences, filling the gap historically created in the historical three-way division between biological/physiological, psychological and social sciences.

References

1. Schrödinger, E. (1944). *What is life?* Cambridge: Cambridge University Press.
2. Von Bertalanffy, L. (1968). *General system theory.* New York: George Braziller.
3. Lane, N. (2015). *The vital question: Energy, evolution, and the origins of complex life.* London: W. W. Norton.
4. Hodges, A. (2014). *Alan Turing: The Enigma.* London: Vintage Books.
5. Mukherjee, S. (2016). *The gene: An intimate history.* New York, NY: Scribner.
6. Ward, P. S., & Thompson, C. B. (2012). Signaling in control of cell growth and metabolism. *Cold Spring Harbor Perspectives in Biology, 4*(7), a006783. https://doi.org/10.1101/cshperspect.a006783.
7. Watson, J. D., & Crick, F. H. C. (1953). A structure for deoxyribose nucleic acid. *Nature, 171*(4356), 737–738.
8. O'Connor, T. & Wong, H.Y. (2015). Emergent Properties. In E.N. Zalta (Ed.), *The Stanford Encyclopedia of Philosophy* (Summer 2015 Edition), URL = <https://plato.stanford.edu/archives/sum2015/entries/properties-emergent/>. Accessed 12/21/2018.

9. Wimsatt, W. C. (2007). *Re-engineering philosophy for limited beings: Piecewise approximations to reality.* Cambridge, MA: Harvard University Press.
10. Bechtel, W., & Richardson, R. C. (2010). *Discovering complexity: Decomposition and localization as strategies in scientific research* (2nd ed.). Cambridge: MIT Press.
11. Falcon, A. (2015). Aristotle on Causality. In E.N. Zalta (Ed.), *The Stanford Encyclopedia of Philosophy* (Spring 2015 Edition), URL = <https://plato.stanford.edu/archives/spr2015/entries/Aristotle-causality/>. Accessed 12/21/2018.
12. Fodor, J. (1997). Special sciences: Still autonomous after all these years. *Philosophical Perspectives, 11,* 149–163.
13. Fodor, J. (1974). Special sciences (Or: The disunity of science as a working hypothesis). *Synthese, 28*(2), 97–115.
14. Putnam, H. (1978). *Meaning and the moral sciences.* London: Routledge & Kegan Paul.
15. van Riel, R., & Van Gulick, R. (2018). Scientific Reduction. In E.N. Zalta (Ed.), *The Stanford Encyclopedia of Philosophy* (Summer 2015 Edition), URL = <https://plato.stanford.edu/archives/sum2018/entries/scientific-reduction/>. Accessed 12/21/2018.
16. Kim, J. (1993). The nonreductivist's troubles with mental causation. In A. M. John Heil (Ed.), *Mental causation* (pp. 189–210). Oxford: Clarenden Press.
17. Robb, D. and Heil, J., "Mental Causation", *The Stanford Encyclopedia of Philosophy* (Winter 2018 Edition), Edward N. Zalta (ed.), URL = <https://plato.stanford.edu/archives/win2018/entries/mental-causation/>. Accessed 12/21/2018.
18. Papineau, D. (2016). Naturalism. In E.N. Zalta (Ed.), *The Stanford Encyclopedia of Philosophy* (Winter 2016 Edition), URL = <https://plato.stanford.edu/archives/win2016/entries/naturalism/>. Accessed 23/06/2017.
19. McLaughlin, B., & Bennett, K. (2018). Supervenience. In E.N. Zalta (Ed.), *The Stanford Encyclopedia of Philosophy* (Winter 2018 Edition), URL = <https://plato.stanford.edu/archives/win2018/entries/supervenience/>. Accessed 12/21/2018.
20. Dasgupta, S. (2014). The possibility of physicalism. *The Journal of Philosophy, 111*(9/10), 557–592.
21. Schaffer, J. (2000). Causation by disconnection. *Philosophy of Science, 67*(2), 285–300.
22. Hall, N. (2002). Non-locality on the cheap? A new problem for counterfactual analyses of causation. *Noûs, 36*(2), 276–294.
23. Hall, N. (2004). Two concepts of causation. In J. Collins, N. Hall, & L. A. Paul (Eds.), *Causation and counterfactuals* (pp. 225–276). Cambridge: The MIT Press.
24. Woodward, J. (2003). *Making things happen: A theory of causal explanation.* New York, NY: Oxford University Press.

25. Mitchell, S. D. (2003). *Biological complexity and integrative pluralism.* Cambridge, MA: Cambridge University Press.
26. Fodor, J. (1987). *Psychosemantics: The problem of meaning in the philosophy of mind.* Explorations in Cognitive Science. Cambridge: The MIT Press.
27. Griffiths, P. E. (2001). Genetic information: A metaphor in search of a theory. *Philosophy of Science, 68*(3), 394–412.
28. Bechtel, W. (2008). *Mental mechanisms: Philosophical perspectives on cognitive neuroscience.* London: Psychology Press.
29. Sargis, M. (2016). *About the endocrine system; Endocrine glands and hormones.* https://www.endocrineweb.com/endocrinology/about-endocrine-system. Accessed August 21, 2017.
30. Engel, G. L. (1977). The need for a new medical model: A challenge for biomedicine. *Science, 196*(4286), 129–136.
31. Engel, G. L. (1987). Foreword. In L. Foss & K. Rothenberg, *The second medical revolution: From biomedicine to infomedicine.* Boston: New Science Library/Shambhala.
32. Foss, L., & Rothenberg, K. (1987). *The second medical revolution: From biomedicine to infomedicine.* Boston: New Science Library/Shambhala.
33. Quirke, V., & Gaudilliere, J. P. (2008). The era of biomedicine: Science, medicine, and public health in Britain and France after the Second World War. *Medical History, 52*(4), 441–452.

CHAPTER 3

Psychology Regulates Activity in the Social World

Abstract Moving on from biology to psychology, we propose that the core function of the psychological is *agency*. This conception of the psychological in the new reworked biopsychosocial theory is consistent with current psychology and neuroscience, for example the so-called 4 Es model of cognition as *embodied*, *embedded*, *enactive* and *extended*. Agency has conditions in the social and political domains—signified by concepts of autonomy and recognition—the failure of which can jeopardise the perception and exercise of agency and hence psychological health. The third component of the biopsychosocial—the social—is defined within this framework as essentially to do with control and distribution of the resources necessary for biological and psychological life. The main theme of biopsychosocial interactions threads through the chapter, including theorising the notorious (for reductionism) 'top-down' causal pathways. This chapter aims to provide a framework to understand how factors involved in health and disease, particularly in the contexts of public health, and managing with long-term conditions, are increasingly seen to extend beyond the internal biological environment into the psychological, social, economic and political conditions of living.

Keywords Agency · Biopsychosocial systems · Embodied cognition · Post-dualism · Social determinants of health · Top-down causation

D. Bolton and G. Gillett,
The Biopsychosocial Model of Health and Disease,
https://doi.org/10.1007/978-3-030-11899-0_3

3.1 The Psychological as Embodied Agency

Mind Is Embodied

The decisive break from dualism in psychological science came with the development of the information-processing paradigm from around the 1960s onwards, in parallel with its development in biology. The paradigm ties together the biological and the psychological. Biology as physiology and anatomy deals with the body inside the skin, while psychology as behavioural science models functioning of the whole organism in its external environment, regulated and controlled by the central nervous system. The complexity of living beings increases massively in phylogenesis and ontogenesis and for human beings in maturity, behavioural science becomes psychology, and the information-processing paradigm is alternatively called the 'cognitive paradigm'. The paradigm shift was gradual: the early cognitive models were not primarily biological, relying on concepts like computation (operations on symbols), and representations, as if of some independent reality already there fixed. Subsequently, the models have become more biological, using models of embodied cognition involved with action [1–3].

Recent developments include 4E cognition [4], which characterises cognition in these four interconnected terms:

1. 'Embodied' (in the body)
2. 'Embedded' (in the environment; in causal loops with it)
3. 'Enactive' (Acting in and manipulating the environment, directly, not via a representation or model; the environment offers affordances, or opportunities, for action and manipulation)
4. 'Extended' (Extended to the body and environment, including devices used for cognitive functioning).

Embodied cognition involves the whole body, is action-based, dynamical, involving feedback loops, comprising sensory inputs, cognition as prediction, affect, decision, motor planning, modification by experience, and so on, all fundamentally in the service of action in the environment. The new approach is biopsychological but the psychological soon merges—along with the biological—into the social, because the environment is for us substantially social. The fundamental connection between cognitive and social processes, involving such as attention, memory and thought, was identified in the 1920s by the psychologist Lev Vygotsky [5]. Social, interpersonal processes pervade the aspects of cognition identified by the new 4E model (e.g. [6]).

This new view of the psychological can be called 'embodied agency' for short. The term captures two ideas that are fundamental themes in the biopsychosocial model being developed here: first, that the 'I' that knows, the psychological, is also (in) an object among others, a biological body; and, second, that the biopsychosocial individual, the person, is an active, causal power. The broad paradigm of embodied agency in the current science constitutes a new view of human nature, replacing the dualism that, while formulated in the seventeenth century, remained with great influence as psychological science emerged in the nineteenth century into the twentieth century. The new approach appeared, as is sometimes the case, earlier in philosophy than in the science. Critical concepts relating cognition to embodiment and action appeared in nineteenth-century post-Kantian philosophy, especially in the so-called phenomenological tradition, with clear, explicit expression by the mid-twentieth century in Maurice Merleau-Ponty's work [7].

The concept of embodied agency is fundamental in the biopsychosocial theory of health and disease. It links physical with psychological health and implicates pathways between them. We will argue that psychological health depends on the development of a viable enough—for the person—sense of agency, such that, if this condition is not met, mental health is jeopardised, and so also, via complex biopsychological pathways, is physical health. The conditions of embodied agency are biopsychosocial; they are drawn out through this chapter and their relevance to health through Chapter 4.

In the new theoretical approach based on the concept of embodied agency, the whole acting body is involved, but the nervous systems have a specific role in processing information, organisation, regulation and control. We quote below descriptions of the several nervous systems, in lay terms for the public, on the website of the Science Museum in London. The quotations, which are under the main heading '*Who am I?*', illustrate the current science moving into culture, and several key interconnected points relevant to the line of thought we are pursuing here: first, that mind and body are thoroughly involved with one another, replacing mind–body dualism; second, that in this context the body is characterised not in mechanical terms, but in terms of functional processes involving information transfer and control; third, that these processes are not limited to the brain, but pervade the several nervous systems and their functional relationships that extend throughout the body and into processes that we do not think of as mental at all (such as digestion and temperature control). In short, mental functioning is entangled with biological functioning. The quotations from the Science Museum as follows [8]:

> What does the central nervous system do? Your spinal cord receives information from the skin, joints and muscles of your body. It also carries the nerves that control all your movements. Your brain is the most complicated part of your nervous system. It receives information directly from your ears, eyes, nose and mouth, as well as from the rest of your body via the spinal cord. It uses this information to help you react, remember, think and plan, and then sends out the appropriate instructions to your body.
>
> What does the peripheral nervous system do? Some of your peripheral nervous system (PNS) is under your voluntary control - the nerves that carry instructions from your brain to your limbs, for example. As well as controlling your muscles and joints, it sends all the information from your senses back to your brain. Other parts of your PNS are controlled by the brain automatically. This is the autonomic nervous system. It manages some things your body does 'without thinking' like digestion and temperature control.
>
> What does the autonomic nervous system do? There are three parts to your autonomic nervous system: 1. The sympathetic system is responsible for your body's 'fight or flight' reaction. 2. The parasympathetic system looks after the workings of your body during rest and recuperation. It also controls your heart rate and body temperature under normal conditions. 3. The enteric system controls the workings of your gut.

The radical shift in thought in this early twenty-first century account of 'Who am I?' compared with Descartes' seventeenth-century answer to the same question in the *Second Meditation* can be readily seen [9] (pp. 75 and 112):

> But what then am I? A thing that thinks. What is a thing which thinks? It is a thing which doubts, understands, affirms, denies, wills, refuses, which also imagines and senses....
>
> Because, on the one side I have a clear and distinct idea of myself, insofar as I am only a thinking and unextended thing, and as, on the other,

> I possess a distinct idea of body, inasmuch it is only an extended and unthinking thing, it is certain that this I… is entirely and absolutely distinct from my body, and can exist without it.

The twenty-first-century version, by contrast, has me and my body entangled together. And, connected, my body is far from 'simply an extended thing'; it is something more able to be a thing that thinks.

One implication of the radical shift from Cartesian dualism to the current science is that neural structures and activities become *a new source of information for models of mental functioning*. Neuroscience is a new third epistemology of mind, adding to the two we already have: recognition of mentality in (the regulation of) behaviour, and introspective reports or declarations. Neuropsychological findings can help shape, for example, the theory of colour vision [10], and models of memory [11] (p. 71). This new epistemology has major application in the theory of the extent to which psychological processes can affect biological processes, interpreting this question as the extent to which central nervous system pathways, especially those associated with modification by voluntary control or practice, affect biological processes. This in turn has application to health-related processes. For example, pain has been shown to be sensitive to central as well as peripheral pathways (to be considered in Chapter 4, Sect. 4.2), while biologically original and fundamental processes such as cell respiration and replication, and their dysfunctions, are probably not, nor the formation and travel of venous thromboembolisms.

The new model of embodied cognition include cognitive psychology and its well-known maxim, used to mark the contrast with behaviourism and unreconstructed conditioning theory, that we respond to the environment as perceived by us, not to stimuli given absolutely. This is a point about human psychology, but there is a broader point that belongs to the information processing paradigm generally, namely, that biological systemic functioning uses information detectors sensitive to specific kinds of signals within a certain range that is relevant to functioning. Biological systems are attuned to particular salient environmental signals, either genetically, or, as a result of learning, as modelled in behavioural learning theory. This is a core working assumption of the new epistemology in the current life and human sciences and accordingly it has multiple linkages. In biology, genetic functioning and environmental interaction are entangled in evolution by natural selection, and ontogenetically in gene environment interactions, to be considered later (Sect. 3.4). Moving to mature human psychology, the topic of the current chapter, the person's perception of reality—whether of themselves, their body and mind, or the world around them including friends and the wider culture—and their responses to it, depend on their interests, needs and values. This epistemology puts the person and their psychology at the centre of the biopsychosocial complex, as the knowing agent, though muddled up with biology and culture. The person is therefore also the centre of attention in biopsychosocial healthcare—a point to be made later in Chapter 4, Sect. 4.2. A specific illustration of the critical role of the person's interpretation of reality came up in Chapter 1, Sect. 1.2, as the epidemiological finding that perception of one's own social status is a better predictor of health outcomes than objectively measured social status. On the other hand, cognitive psychology and the new epistemology of which it is part is not 'idealist'. This is to say: it does not suppose that reality is only appearance. The new epistemology does not have reality as something 'behind' appearance, however, likely to be unknowable, but rather as appearance that is independent of our control. Reality makes itself well-known to us as events beyond our control which seriously impinge on our perceptions, needs and values; such as, serious losses, accidents, war, illness and impending death. Another aspect of the same point links with misperception and epistemological disorder. While we have latitude on how we represent reality we do not have a free hand, and if we go too far adrift in tracking it, we are potentially exposed to harm, and if and when we persist we are cognitively incompetent or in denial, and as more harm accrues, in a mental health condition. In the new philosophical framework, the ontology and epistemology of appearance and reality can be run in terms that overlap with health and disease.

Agency Is Causal

Nervous systems regulate internal and external behaviour. Central nervous systems have a super-status, though un-omnipotent, controlling other regulatory systems and behaviour as a whole, and all this reaches its peak in the human central nervous system, the largest and most complex, with highly developed specialised cortical areas and connections with so-called 'executive' functions. This from The University of California website [12]:

> The term "Executive functions" refers to the higher-level cognitive skills you use to control and coordinate your other cognitive abilities and behaviors. The term is a business metaphor, where the chief executive monitors all of the different departments so that the company can move forward as efficiently and effectively as possible. Who we are, how we organize our lives, how we plan and how we then execute those plans is largely guided by our executive system.
>
> Executive functions can be divided into organizational and regulatory abilities. Organization includes gathering information and structuring it for evaluation. Regulation involves evaluating the available information and modulating your responses to the environment.... The executive system involves the prefrontal cortex, basal ganglia and thalamus... The frontal lobes are the last areas of the brain to fully develop. This area of the brain was evolutionarily late to appear and is much larger in human beings than in our closest non-human primate relatives. The frontal lobes typically account for about 40% of the human brain.

Self-regulation is one aspect of the causal power of agency among several, all entangled. Most plainly, embodied agency interacts with other physical things; it cannot act at all without supporting ground; the body as a physical thing, using the skeletal muscular system, can move other physical things, and is moved by other physical things. All these interactions involve energy transfer according to Newton's laws. The behaviour of the skeletal muscular system towards goals in relation to the environment and the effects of on-going behaviour is *self-regulated*, involving the nervous systems and executive functioning specifically, as above. Further, our activity in the social environment involves *inter-regulation*, this interspersed with physical interactions between us, benign or harmful. These themes of agency, inter-agency and causation run through the biopsychosocial in health, disease, security and injury, and hence they appear explicitly or implicitly throughout this book.

A recently proposed and influential philosophical theory of causation, the so-called 'interventionist' theory—see, for example, James Woodward [13]—emphasises linkage between *causation* and *agency*, consistent with what is suggested here. The interventionist approach emphasises that our interests in causal connections and explanations are linked to our practical concerns of being able reliably to bring about changes. At the same time the interventionist approach is aligned with experimental methodology, especially its technological implications: if A causes B, we can manipulate B by manipulating A. Thus it has application across the sciences. The practical, technological emphasis of the interventionist approach to causation is particularly well suited to identifying specific, localised causal connections in complex systems, as opposed to causal connections covered by general laws, and has been developed more in connection with biology and neuroscience than physics. Particularly relevant to a core theme in this book, the interventionist approach can accommodate causation by regulatory mechanisms, including explanations involving non-events, of the sort considered in Chapter 2, Sect. 2.2.

Embodiment Involves Intersubjectivity

The Cartesian philosophy and its legacy was fundamentally solipsistic in the sense of envisaging only a single, unique subjectivity. It was not, at its foundations, social. The Cartesian ego, divorced from the body, never could know another subjectivity like itself: all the Cartesian ego could ever come across were objects of one sort or another; mechanical things in nature, including the body, or else perceptions in the mind—but it never could encounter as an object of knowledge another knowing subject like itself. For another subject to be an object of knowledge, subjectivity has to be something in the world that is known—that is, embodied. The dismantling of the seventeenth-century materialist-dualist thought framework involves not only embodiment of subjectivity, but intersubjectivity: the social assumes a foundational role. Embodiment and intersubjectivity make an appearance in philosophy following Kant in Fichte and Hegel: the knowing 'subject' becomes the human being, down to earth, as opposed to being disembodied, transcendental (outside of material, space and time)—and as such it is able to recognise another like itself (see, e.g., [14]). The foundational linkage in post-dualism between the biological body, knowing subjectivity and the social, becoming then moral and political, all with implications for the theory of health and disease, threads through these middle sections of this essay.

> Inter-subjectivity opens up whole new aspects of regulatory control and communication. It involves interaction, between bodies and minds, involving both energy-exchanges and information-exchanges. We do not exchange information with the natural, inanimate environment: the flow of information is one-way, from it inwards to us; we do not send information to it to influence it; it has no information receptors or processing

mechanisms; no systems functioning towards ends. In the social environment, however, all this changes, another aspect of the interpenetration of the psychological and the social.

3.2 Biopsychosocial Conditions of Agency

The Concept of Agency Has Broad Scope

Agency as the fundamental post-dualist concept spins off in many directions, with many alternative or related names; it threads through and criss-crosses the sciences and humanities: biology and neuroscience, psychology and its many subdivisions, especially social and developmental psychology, the philosophy of language and moral theory, social science and politics. The title of this section 'conditions of agency' refers in all these directions. We do not aim to review the science or the philosophy, but, consistent with the method so far, to clarify the conceptual and scientific foundations of the theory which replaces physicalism, dualism and reductionism, and which is required to underpin the biopsychosocial model of health and disease. As indicated, these foundations turn out to involve much more than biology.

Biopsychological Preconditions and Implications

Agency requires brain maturation and skill acquisition through infancy and childhood to adolescence, addressed in the increasingly intertwined developmental psychology and developmental neuroscience literatures (e.g. [15]). Subjectively, alongside and interacting with practical competence, with complex neuropsychological underpinnings, we develop the experience of agency. Here, for example, the beginning of a paper by Synofzik and colleagues presenting a general model of the experience of agency as based in an interplay between prediction and postdiction [16] (p. 1):

> The experience of agency, i.e., the registration that I am the initiator of my actions, is a basic and constant underpinning of our interaction with the world: whenever we grasp, type, or walk, we register the resulting sensory consequences as caused by ourselves.

Here can be seen from another perspective the tight link between agency and self-causation. And as always in regulatory and control processes, there is the possibility of error; one of the applications of the research programme on the sense of agency is to some of the signs and symptoms associated with the diagnosis of schizophrenia.

A new field in neuroscience is the development of the social brain in adolescence, interwoven with increasing executive functioning. This abstract from a review article by Sarah-Jayne Blakemore and Suparna Choudhury [17] (p. 296):

> Adolescence is a time of considerable development at the level of behaviour, cognition and the brain. This article reviews histological and brain imaging studies that have demonstrated specific changes in neural architecture during puberty and adolescence, outlining trajectories of grey and white matter development. The implications of brain development for executive functions and social cognition during puberty and adolescence are discussed. Changes at the level of the brain and cognition may map onto behaviours commonly associated with adolescence. Finally, possible applications for education and social policy are briefly considered.

The concept of 'agency' also appears as 'self-determination' in the theory of that name proposed by Edward Deci and Richard Ryan, social and clinical psychologists. Here, for example, [18] (pp. 227):

> Self-determination theory (SDT) maintains that an understanding of human motivation requires a consideration of innate psychological needs for competence, autonomy, and relatedness… Social contexts and individual differences that support satisfaction of the basic needs facilitate natural growth processes including intrinsically motivated behavior and integration of extrinsic motivations, whereas those that forestall autonomy, competence, or relatedness are associated with poorer motivation, performance, and well-being.

The linkage of self-determination to psychological needs and to well-being is the direction we are pursuing here. What we are proposing for the biopsychosocial model also has many points in common with Albert Bandura's social cognitive theory of agency [19, 20].

Language an Instrument of Agency

Information transfer is essentially involved with regulation; it pervades biological functioning, and equally pervades behavioural relations within species. Language is one of our human within-species signalling systems; we use it to let each know the current state of dynamical play, for reporting, and to influence one another, as command. It is an expression and an instrument of agency. At the same time as being inherently social, language is also the means of much of our thinking, our psychology, another aspect of the interpenetration of the psychological and the social. Much twentieth-century theory of language has worked its way around such points. Here, for example, one of the pioneers, Lev Vygotsky, the developmental psychologist, writing in the early 1930s [21] (pp. 69–70):

> Children master the social forms of behaviour and transfer these forms to themselves… The validity of this law is nowhere more obvious than in the use of the sign. A sign is always originally a means used for social purposes, a means of influencing others, and only later becomes a means of influencing oneself. … If we want to clarify genetically the origins of the voluntary function of the word and why the word overrides motor responses, we must inevitably arrive at the real function of commanding in both ontogenesis and phylogenesis.

The philosopher Ludwig Wittgenstein developed a new philosophy of language from around the 1930s based on action and communication. His *Philosophical Investigations* starts with examples of people cooperating and communicating when shopping and building [22] (paras. 1, 2 and 8), and comments in paragraphs 18–19:

> Do not be troubled by the fact that languages (2) and (8) consist only of orders… It is easy to imagine a language consisting only of orders and reports in battle.—Or a language consisting only of questions and expressions for answering yes and no. And innumerable others.——And to imagine a language means to imagine a form of life.

In this context, the key question in Wittgenstein's philosophy of language becomes: *what does it mean to follow a rule?*—a topic closely linked to the concept of *regulation* that permeates current biological and behavioural sciences. The conclusion to Wittgenstein's analysis has rule-following in language closely linked with agreement in practice [22] (paras. 240–242). In biological inter-regulatory systems, the concord is set up by selective pressure over evolutionary timescales.

Agency as Moral Responsibility

A strand in moral theory examines the logic and purpose of attributing moral responsibility (scc, c.g., [23]). There are debates as to whether this presupposes free will, genuine self-determination, and in what sense, and debates as to whether praise and blame are made on merits, a matter of what is deserved, or as a means to influence the other. The first consideration links with further moral concepts, bringing in notions of justice, for example, while the second—attributing moral responsibility as means of influencing each other—highlights processes with direct connection to our current themes. Instructions or exhortations from one to another are backed up, if the necessary power asymmetries are in place, by moral sanctions, praise or blame, and these social-moral mechanisms of control, more or less benign, are internalised as we acquire prosocial behaviour.

In short, as agency interpenetrates the social it becomes involved with morality. The moral emotions such as shame and guilt, conversely feelings of self-worth, are fundamental to our psychological life, and when the negative emotions of self-blame become barely controllable, they figure prominently in health conditions. Attribution of illness involves excuse from blame, but also carries risk of suspicion and exclusion, issues taken up in the next chapter (Sect. 4.2). All these things involve much more than our biology and in the new biopsychosocial theory they are all relevant to health and disease.

Agency as Autonomy Is a High Political Value

Psychological agency merges into *political autonomy*. 'Autonomy' in the Greek refers to self-legislation. The term was applied originally in politics to self-governing states as opposed to colonies, was later employed in moral theory by Immanuel Kant in the high Enlightenment, becoming fundamental to liberal political philosophy [24]. Discussion of the various uses and meanings of autonomy which criss-cross the psychological and the political, and their relevance to the concept of mental disorder can be found in [25]. The concept of autonomy is also prominent in bioethics,, affirming the right of the person in medical contexts to exercise control over what is done to his or her body, linking moral and legal rights with our biology [26]. The concept is also used in theorising the social gradient in health, referred to in Sect. 2.1. For example, Michael Marmot argues that 'it is not simply position in the hierarchy that accounts for worse health among individuals of lower status … but what position in the hierarchy means for what one can do in a given society: the degree of autonomy and social participation' [27] (p. 1306).

Brain development of adolescents related to executive and social functioning was referred to above, and reappears here as the development of psychological and political autonomy. The adolescent becoming adult is recognised as an independent citizen, capable of work and contracts and childcare, for example, with assumption of moral and legal responsibility. These processes run across sectors and scientific disciplines—illustrating how split-up sciences and policies have to work together to grasp the development of the biopsychosocial being—and they all impinge on aspects of adolescent health problems—on risks, management and recovery.

Agency/Autonomy Depend on Recognition

Agency in interpersonal and political activity depends on the person as agent being recognised as such. There is a close linkage between embodied, active cognition and intersubjectivity in post-Kantian philosophy, noted above Sect. 3.1, and intersubjectivity is interwoven with the recognition problem. Hegel has a famous passage in the *Phenomenology of Spirit* on the meeting of two people and processes of mutual recognition [28] (pp. 86ff.). He develops a complex argument to the effect that recognition of the other is essential to the development of self and self-consciousness, and it may well be that something of that sort is correct. The context in Hegel is the philosophical project of absolute knowledge that for present purposes was transitional and is irrelevant. The application here is that the philosophical foundations of biopsychology include social *recognition* as necessary for the development and exercise of agency. Recognition involves social power balances. In Hegel, the appearance of the concept is immediately politicised, with argument to the effect that recognition is impossible in the 'lordship–bondage' or 'master–slave' relationship. Subsequently, the concept has been used in political philosophy to theorise the dynamics between more and less powerful groups (e.g. [29–31]).

In benign, caring social groups, with participating members well enough disposed towards one another—functional families, kinship structures, cohesive communities—people recognise one another: they know how to respect each other's agency, albeit within socially proscribed rules and regulations, how to care for, educate, provide opportunities and cultivate voice and practice in children. In short, inclusive communities provide conditions for agency, albeit subject to its rules. If however such communities are excluded from access to resources by more powerful forces, community and individual autonomy is threatened, raising risk of ill health at both levels. These issues are taken up in the next section.

3.3 The Socio-Political: Who Gets to Control What?

Regulatory Control of Biopsychosocial Resources

The 'social' is the third component of the triumvirate invoked by the Biopsychosocial Model as relevant to health and disease, and we turn now to consider it. However, we have already had to start this in the preceding section on the psychological as agency. Because agency involves exercise of power, it is highly sensitive to uses and abuses of power, to the political. Social processes are approached in the social sciences directly however, not via the psychological as agency, but similar themes appear either way round.

The subject matter of the social sciences can be described in terms of social structures, functions, organisation and regulation. This is consistent with the view proposed here that these and related concepts and principles are found throughout the biopsychosocial. Two main themes in the social domain are *group cohesion* and *allocation of resources*, and both are implicated in models of health and disease. As considered at the end of the last section, cohesive communities such as kinship structures can provide conditions for agency, subject to their rules and regulations. We turn here to consider the theme of distribution and allocation of resources.

The distribution of resources, prioritising among needs, prioritising between recipients, is a fundamental feature of social groups, from families to the state. It is a vast elaboration of the sort of distributive, prioritising processes already apparent in basic biological control systems, the delivery of chemicals necessary for Krebs' cycle, for example, and the control of metabolic processes by the nervous system. Control mechanisms that up- or down-regulate resource allocation are causal:

they make a difference to what happens. In the social world, a general word for this kind of causal control is 'power'. Distributive and prioritising functions are defined by socio-economic rules and regulations, backed up by state or non-state power, with sanctions involving the use of force and the deprivation of autonomy and liberty. The exercise of power is one defining characteristic of *politics*, and in this sense 'the social' in biopsychosocial theory applied to health, to do with the distribution of resources, is essentially 'the political'. The highly influential political scientist Harold Lasswell clearly identified this point decades ago, and one of his major works has the title: *Politics: Who Gets What, When, How* [32].

Resources needed for biological health include—no surprises here—access to energy-related provisions, such as food, clean water, shelter to help maintain body temperature, at minimum, extending to healthy diet and exercise opportunities. As the biomedical sciences have understood progressively more detail of our internal biology, so our biological requirements have become more understood. These requirements are basically met by the environment, and as the environmental sciences have understood progressively more about environmental conditions, local and global, so our environmental requirements have become more understood, along with threats. All these well-worked areas are signalled here as part of the biological-environmental-social-psychological whole picture, and to make the uncontroversial point that socio-political processes regulate and control distribution of physical, chemical and biological resources, according to wealth and wealth differences or alternatively according to principles of social justice. The more access to resources, at the individual or population level, the lower the risk of disease. The same point reappears post-onset. The more wealthy a person or state, the sooner healthcare can be accessed, the better the detection and treatment, and the better chance of favourable outcome. All this is well-known and well-understood. We focus more on the more recently recognised and less well theorised causal interplay between socio-political control of processes affecting psychological health—and hence, via that pathway, biological health.

As argued so far, social structures can cultivate agency or they can inhibit it. If a person or group controls the action of another person or group, they so far fail to recognise the agency of the other, and tend to control the interaction in such a way as to disqualify it. Agency can be denied by various processes of psychosocial exclusion: if a person is not noticed, not consulted, not listened to, has no place at the table when important decisions affecting them are being made—then, so far, they have no opportunity for agency in the social group. Options collapse: to withdrawal from free action, to doing only what is prescribed by more powerful others—typically under threat of sanctions for disobedience and disruption, sanctions typically involving brute, physical–biological force. Conversely, when agency is recognised, insofar as the person is allowed and encouraged to have their voice and to influence affairs, agency is realised. This intersubjective relationality can be expressed by saying, somewhat paradoxically, that one cannot be an autonomous agent all by oneself, a point emphasised in feminist theory [33].

Social exclusion has been explored more in political philosophy and related social theory than in psychology. We referred previously to Hegel's theory of recognition and just above to feminist theory. Other relevant active literatures are critical race theory (e.g. [34]), and postcolonial studies (e.g. [35]). Related philosophical theory includes Miranda Fricker's important new concept of 'epistemic injustice' [36] and the related notion of 'epistemic violence' (e.g. [37]). The core idea is that a person's epistemic status—their status as a knowing agent—can be undermined and disqualified by prejudicial use of power. The role of epistemic disqualification in theorising health risks has still to be worked out.

Social exclusion mechanisms involve micro-interpersonal and macrosocial interactions that can operate at any or all points in the lifespan. Others relate specifically to access to resources and opportunities necessary for development of agency in children. Agency requires the development of knowledge and skills and therefore depends on access to and quality of education and training, in turn typically linked to privileged group membership. Socio-economic-political power structures keep a tight hold on distribution of education and training resources, and this is another factor—along with and interwoven with distribution of biological resources—that maintains linkage between wealth and health. Greater access to education and training tends towards greater employment prospects and hence greater social status and wealth, creating a benign circle; and conversely. This is part of the biopsychosocial background of the so-called 'social gradient of health', reviewed below in Sect. 2.1, a linking mechanism being chronic stress, to be considered in Chapter 4, Sect. 4.3.

Socio-Political Causes Really Are Causes

The arguments so far are relevant to disputes in epidemiology regarding the causal status of the social determinant of health. In the reductionist world picture, only physical–chemical biological causes are real, while psychological and social causes are chimerical. In this picture, associations between poverty and poor health could be explained in terms of biological processes such as poor diet, hygiene or smoke inhalation, while social factors are something else, kind of causal, but not really, because not biological. The social factors appear less like causes, more like delivery or exposure processes, as opposed to the really causal biochemical or microbiological mechanisms—all these thoughts summed up in the idea that social factors are not real causes but something else, perhaps 'distal risks'. The counter-argument developed here is that delivery and differential exposure processes are equally causal, apparent already at the basic biological level. The problem and counter-argument in more detail as follows.

Here is William Cockerham in his book *Social Causes of Health and Disease* [38] (p. 1; citations omitted):

> Stress, poverty, low socio-economic status, unhealthy lifestyles, and unpleasant living and work conditions are among the many inherently social variables typically regarded by laypersons as causes of ill health. However, with the exception of stress, this view is not expressed in much of the research literature… Usually social variables are characterised as distant or secondary influences on health and illness, not as direct causes. Being poor, for example, is held to produce greater exposure to something that will make a person sick, rather than bring on sickness itself…

Other epidemiological theorists have echoed this complaint, for example, Kelly and colleagues [39] (p. 310):

> The importance of behavioural and social factors notwithstanding, they seldom find their way into etiological discussions of mechanisms of causation, instead being merely defined as risks or risk factors.

This is a major issue in the epidemiological literature. In her important paper on epidemiology and causation, Nancy Krieger [40] argued that while the epidemiological literature since the 1960s has recognised complex multifactorial causation, it became preoccupied with statistical modelling, without developing an adequate theory of causation. In a later paper Krieger argues, consistent with the views proposed here, that power—power over and power to do—structures people's engagement with the world and their exposures to material and psychosocial health hazards, driving health inequities, and that power does not readily map onto a metric of proximal or distal [41].

A related issue is whether apparent social causes are really confounded by biological causes. Here is Michael Marmot, discussing this issue, arguing that social factors, and a biopsychosocial model, have to be invoked to explain the social gradient in biological health risks [42] (p. 43):

> Coming back to the Whitehall study, people had the idea that if we could explain the gradient in CHD [coronary heart disease] mortality by cholesterol, then social class would not be causal. I think this is too simplistic, because social class can determine the cholesterol level… In fact, mean plasma cholesterol in the first Whitehall study was marginally higher in the top grades and in the Whitehall II study there was essentially no difference by grade of employment. In both studies there was a very clear social gradient in smoking.
>
> This comes back to asking the question of why we need a Biopsychosocial Model if we have smoking? An important psychosocial question is why is there a social gradient in smoking? It is not enough to know that smoking causes disease. We need to know why it is in the UK as a whole, close to 100% of women and 80% of men in the most deprived category are smokers…

In the terms of the view proposed here, the causal status of social determinants of health has seemed problematic because of a mistaken conception of causation, limited to biology, but biology presumed to be a matter of physics and chemistry, and therefore quite unlike social mechanisms that deliver health resources or toxins to exposed populations. Once understanding of biological causal explanation is updated in line with the biological and biomedical science of the past few decades, it can be seen to comprise not only physics and chemistry, but also and in very large part specification of mechanisms that organise and deliver resources all around internal biological systems, and which remove toxins, or fail to; and further, those internal distribution processes are entirely dependent on what can be taken in from the external environment, clean air and healthy diet, for example, or the opposites, in which case any social mechanisms such as social inclusion and exclusion that affect availability of health-promoting resources or exposure to toxins are very much part of the causal chain, whether distal or otherwise.

As Marmot implies in the above quote, we need a broader biopsychosocial model to comprehend social causal processes as well as and interacting with biological causal pathways. Such a model also brings into view the psychological and its relation to the social, including distribution of resources that promote development and exercise of agency, such as education, employment, and social cohesion that can cultivate agency. Insofar as societies are organised so that these are not available to particular groups, the individuals in those groups are at raised risk of psychological health difficulties as well as physical health difficulties, and either way this social risk raising is causal.

The statistical modelling of multifactorial causal interactions, especially in non-linear systems involving feedback/feedforward effects over time, presents challenges in epidemiology. Galea and colleagues [43] examine the issues in the case of 'the cause of obesity', listing seven broad headings of types of relevant factor, each with many specifics, from genes and gene expression through to national food and agriculture policy, with many individual, neighbourhood and social levels in-between. The authors note, consistent with the view proposed here, that higher level social factors are indeed causal, and go onto to consider the counterfactual approach to identifying a single modifiable causal factor, and the use of multilevel regression modelling of multiple risks. They note, however, the limitation of regression to capture non-linear effects of the outcome dependent variable(s) on the independent variables, and propose use of complex systems dynamic computational models which can take into account not only risks at multiple levels but also interrelations between them.

The topic of this section, social causation, is a long-standing major topic in the social sciences. The hermeneutic tradition, which defined social processes, meaning and understanding, as separate from causal explanation of nature by physics and chemistry, as outside nature and causation altogether, was briefly discussed in Chapter 1, Sect. 1.3. The hermeneutic approach is also consistent with emphasising that individual psychology and action underpins social phenomena, a view associated with Max Weber and known as 'methodological individualism' in the social sciences (for review see, e.g., [44]). Another tradition, from Émile Durkheim, proposes that the subject matter of the social sciences are distinctive social facts and causal processes. This kind of approach, sometimes called 'methodological holism' (for review see, e.g., [45]), can be seen as opposed to methodological holism, requiring reconciliation between the two views. For example, List and Spiekermann [46] propose reconciliation using concepts from current analytical philosophy of mind, such as 'supervenience'. Our approach to the relation between individual level and social level causal explanation is part of the general theory of biopsychosocial systems outlined in the next section.

3.4 General Theory of Biopsychosocial Systems

The Thread so Far

We pick up here the line of thought developing a general model of biopsychosocial ontology and interactions that was set up at the end of Chapter 1, Sect. 1.3. Throughout the chapters so far, the ontology and the theory of causation have been of a piece. The key principle in the ontology starts with the relation of biology to the physics and chemistry of matter. Within the constraints of energy equations, complex molecular structures form, capable of regulating energetic processes, especially increasing energy differences, running counter to the second law of thermodynamics, temporarily, though replicating in the meantime. Thus the ontology blurs into causal theory: different complex dynamical forms have different causal properties. This was the line of thought in the first part of Chapter 2. In the second part, the contrast was drawn with the limited, uniform, flat ontology of physicalism, which, in its most coherent form, would envisage only physical causation, but, faced with apparently valid causal principles in the psychological and social sciences, principles able to predict, retreats to the physicalist ontological claim only, admitting psychological and social causation, though inevitably has trouble theorising these additional causes without additional ontology. Now that we have in this third chapter so far proposed an account of the psychological and social, we can now generalise the points made in connection with biology to the psychological and the social.

Life Forms: Diversity Amidst the Physics

The idea proposed in Chapter 2 that biological forms and ends proliferate within 'free spaces' permitted by physics energy equations carries through to the biopsychosocial. As a rule, nothing in psychology or social science textbooks is ever going to contradict textbooks about human biological systems, and insofar as psychology has any invariants, they will be preserved in the social sciences. There are constraints, but they leave scope for variety. In this sense, psychology exploits biological indeterminacy, for example, in the individual differences that arise partly by genetic constitution and partly by individual learning experiences, expressed as individual choice and agency. Following the same line of thought, social processes elaborate diversity in the biological and the psychological, giving rise to many forms of practice around our biological nature and around agency, intersubjectivity and recognition. The transition from the biological to the psychological and the social is characterised by the appearance of new free spaces in which can arise the twin phenomena of *new forms of organisation* and *diversity and with them new causal processes.* Once we move above physics and chemistry into biology, hence into psychological and social processes, the causation involves information-exchange, communication, regulation and control.

The Logic of Top-Down Causation

There are many kinds of causal pathways in biopsychosocial systems. They can be top-down, bottom-up, and within-levels; they can involve regulatory mechanisms, disruptions to regulatory mechanisms, or have nothing to do with regulation, involving energy exchanges only. Already the abstract picture is complex, even before the specifics, and the contrast is with the single sort of causation envisaged by physicalism, energy transformations covered by a handful of equations.

Traditionally top-down causation has appeared as the most conceptually problematic, disallowed by physicalist reductionism, and behind that, by energy conservation constraints. The problem is relieved when causal processes involving regulation are acknowledged. In this kind of causation, the regulating mechanism and the processes regulated are in the same ontological space—signified exactly by the fact that they interact. In this sense, while we can say that the regulating mechanism is at a 'higher' level than the processes being regulated, this no longer has the connotation that belonged to the concept of level in reductionism, namely that lower levels are ontologically more basic than higher levels. A core principle is that control mechanisms *can up- and down-regulate processes at a 'lower' level, but cannot change their conformity to the lower level laws*. We considered this point in relation to biology, physics and chemistry in the second chapter, but it has some application throughout. In the case of the psychological, our biology gives us both capacity and choice—we have control over our limbs all being well, and some choice between courses of action—but we cannot alter our basic physics, biochemistry or biology: if the rope breaks we fall, if the biological mechanisms controlling cell replication breakdown we cannot by act of will put them right; we survive practically no time without oxygen. Equally, forms of social organisation can vary, but they cannot alter our biology; for example, there are many ways in which social groups organise themselves around death, but they cannot alter the fact, even if we freely imagine life after, or postpone it as long as possible by medical treatments. Or again, forms of social organisation can promote education and training of individuals, but there are limits to achievements deriving from common and individual biopsychology; and forms of social organisation deal with agency and recognition of the individual in the social group in diverse ways, but cannot alter our need for it.

The point that higher level processes can up- or down-regulate lower-level processes, but cannot change the causal laws or principles at the lower level, is clearest at the lowest level, physics and chemistry, where the energy equations never change. As we move away from the physical/chemical laws, however, we never encounter inviolability again. As we move into biology, psychology, and social processes, there is increasing scope for higher level processes not only to up- and down-regulate, but also to affect the lower-level processes themselves, because these lower-level processes are themselves regulatory, not fixed laws of nature. There are some hard and fast rules, but blurred boundaries. For example, there is a boundary, but a blurred one, between biological processes that we can psychologically control—or can learn to control—and those we can't, and a blurred boundary between psychological processes that can be socially controlled, and those that can't. Once we move up from the inviolable laws of physics and chemistry—up from their mathematical equations—the new forms of organisation and principles governing change have themselves a changeable quality.

Biopsychosocial top-down causation is possible because the various systems are all in the same ontological space. Systemic top-down causation always involves agents at the lower level, where the difference is being made, but those agents at the lower level function in ways deriving from their communication- or information-based relationships with wider organizational/regulatory systems. Hormones are biochemicals like the processes they regulate, but their messenger function derives from the state of the brain or other organ that regulates their secretion, and that in turn on states of distant parts of the body. Social authority is imposed on individuals by other individuals, by virtue of their office, a complex idea that includes acceptance of the rules by all parties involved, and the power of the office to force compliance. Causation by regulatory control is not ethereal and mysterious: it involves interaction with the regulated processes by things of the same type, in the same ontological space, but those linked to wider contexts and dynamic relationships.

Psychological regulation of biological processes appears as the alternative to the irredeemably problematic Cartesian problem how immaterial mind could affect the material body. In post-dualist science, mental functioning is embodied, and the central nervous system regulates not only some internal functioning but also goal-directed behaviour in the environment. All of the processes occur in the same ontological space: stimuli are material forms, as are nervous system responses, as are behavioural responses. These forms exercise regulatory control over one another using information-exchange. Specification of a mechanism is specification of the intervening links, in terms of information exchange, up-/down-regulation of subsystemic responses, or whole behaviour responses, and/or in terms of the materials, such as neurons, neuronal assemblies, genes and hormones. Within this paradigm, with the concepts so constructed and ordered, specification of mind–body mechanisms is a scientific task—not a conceptually insoluble problem.

Social regulation of individual, psychological/behavioural processes has the same logic as psychological regulation of biological processes. Social and psychological/behavioural processes occur in the same ontological space; a military officer is a person like the private soldier. The question arises what are the causal properties of the individual person—as opposed to those of the office. Some causal properties of the individual are the same whatever social system they are in, biopsychological properties, let's call them, but others are by virtue of their office within a socially defined and regulated institution, realised in patterns of relationships and causal power within the wider social institution. Only by reference to the wider social institution is it possible to explain why the military officer can control the behaviour of the private soldier. All this is obvious enough; it is not ontologically mysterious. The appearance of mystery is only in the context of reductionism. Away from the reductionist picture, there is nothing ontologically mysterious about social institutions or their causal powers. An adequate explanation of why, for example, a military officer can do what he or she does, involves reference to the long-standing institution of the military, with its accumulated rules and regulations, to the training of the individual person within and by those institutions, and to their appointment as an officer, bringing with it access to power that far exceeds biopsychological nature understood as without institutionally defined office. Apart from causal power, membership of particular social groupings may affect individual psychological/behavioural dispositions. For example, members of disadvantaged groups lacking education are more likely to have lower health literacy and less timely access to healthcare. There can also be associations and possibly causal connections between social phenomena, for example, between state or non-state actors, or between socio-economic class and health outcomes, as evidenced in the social gradient in health. All such relations involve individuals, but some of their causal properties, both what they affect and what they are affected by, depends as much or more on socially defined position than on individual characteristics and differences. This general approach defuses the tension between individual level and social level explanations considered at the end of the previous section.

Biopsychosocial systems work by complex regulatory control mechanisms that are vulnerable to break down. At the same time, biopsychosocial systems tend to self-preservation for as long as possible, which, since the threat of breakdown is ever present, requires a special dedicated class of regulatory mechanisms that protect, disrupt, repair and restore—all more or less successfully. Study of such defensive and maintenance mechanisms take up substantial parts of biomedical and psychological textbooks, and there are social science analogues regarding mechanisms for maintaining social order.

Cross-Disciplinarity and New Human Sciences

The biopsychosocial/environmental whole can be divided up three or four ways, four to include the natural as well as the social environment, using distinctive methodologies to answer distinctive kinds of questions, and then much subdivided in the division of scientific labour. However, the signal from the changes in the life and human sciences reviewed here is increasing need for cross-disciplinarity. The biopsychosocial systems theory approach makes interdependency of the four kinds of phenomena fundamental, especially in modelling real-life problem areas. There is simply too much going on for one disciplinary approach alone. For example, biomedicine restricted to inner organs and systems will not attend much to the psychological attitude of the patient or their social and broad environmental context. The multifactorial and cross-disciplinary nature of the causes of variance in health outcomes also appears in the broad cross-sectoral range of interlinked outcomes, for example, links between health inequalities and educational inequalities (e.g. [27]).

In recognition of the need for cross-disciplinary approaches to problem-solving, they are increasingly encouraged by research funding bodies. For example, there is a new UK cross-research council strategy for mental health, which announces itself like this [47] (p. 1):

> The Research Councils… collectively have an interest in mental health research from a medical, biological, environmental, cultural, societal, technical and historical perspective. We have worked together to develop a cross-disciplinary research agenda, to articulate opportunities for cross-disciplinary working.

The stronger signal from these developments however is that the old headings of sciences which gives the Biopsychosocial Model its name are themselves problematic, especially insofar as they still contain lingering presumptions and prejudices from the old divided spaces, and what is in progress is a biopsychosocial/environmental transdisciplinary revamp across the life and human sciences. It is as if we shouldn't really be starting where we are now, with biology, psychology and social science as separate from one another. These old sciences need reconceptualising so as to manage biopsychosocial and natural environment interactions. A further implication is that new, large scale scientific paradigms will involve these interactions as foundational.

This point applies to the two new, progressive sciences, mostly applied to health and disease: genetics and neuroscience. These two new sciences effectively break down previous categories of biological, psychological, environmental and social—they do not start with these four 'levels' of reality or causal explanation, but rather with an assumption more like bio-environmental-psycho-social integrity. Neuroscience works with a systemic view of the brain, essentially engaged in regulation and control of within-body processes and behaviour in the outer environment, implementing psychological processes, including substantial resources for social processing, while at the same time being biological, neurochemical, genetically influenced; and so on. The new genetics is plainly biopsychosocial, envisaging biological genetic influences, individual differences and social factors, among other environmental factors, as all involved in determination of phenotypes, including health outcomes. The most recently developing field of epigenetics illustrates these features most explicitly and some points are detailed below.

Epigenetic processes are potentially heritable changes in genetic effects on a phenotype that do not involve changes to the underlying DNA sequence. The genome itself is not altered, but specific genes can be expressed, i.e. can be active in the production of proteins, or they can be switched off and inactive—this altering downstream functioning in the internal or external environment. Proximate epigenetic mechanisms include DNA methylation and stable chromatin modifications, and the wider systemic picture has many factors capable of altering these epigenetic mechanisms, including other genes, biological clocks, and exposure to specific external environments. The concept of gene–environment interaction is grounded somewhat differently in molecular genetics and behavioural genetics, corresponding to their distinctive objects of study, concepts and methodologies. In molecular genetics, gene–environment interactions can be understood as effects of specific environmental exposures on gene expression, as above. Measuring gene–environment interactions is methodologically complex, requiring assessment of each component and causal role separately (e.g. [48, 49]). In behavioural genetics, the concept refers to differential phenotypic effects of the same environmental exposure on different genotypes, indexed by statistical interaction in the model.

Epigenetic mechanisms are biologically deep, found already in, for example, plants regulating responses to stress [50]. They appear in animals, the environment for mammals typically including maternal behaviour or other complex social interactions with con-specifics (e.g. [51]; [52]). Epigenetic factors have also been implicated in humans and human diseases, for example, in hypothalamic–pituitary–adrenal function [53] coronary heart disease [54], and in the social gradient of health [55].

A striking illustration of the interpenetration of biological, environmental and psychological processes is the possibility that individual agency qualifies the gene/environment dichotomy. It has been a startling finding in human behavioural genetics that environmental exposures, specifically adverse life events or risks, far from being all independent accidents, are sometimes themselves 'heritable'. Such gene–environment correlations seem to cast doubt on purely environmental causal effects. However, there is a more radical implication here. In their review of gene–environment (G × E) interaction Manuck and McCaffery have this [56] (pp. 62–63):

> An interaction confounded by rGe [gene-environment correlation] might well seem to lack the implications of a true G × E finding. Yet what is the implication, if not confirming a proposition predicated on a frayed dichotomy?... In view of the extent of demonstrated rGE, it seems reasonable to assume that most dimensions of measured experience will have both environmental and genetic determinants, and most G × E studies will not be able to partition genetic and environmental influences on their environmental moderators... Relinquishing pure G × E interaction as the grail of G × E research may encourage interest in a broader expanse of potential gene-exposure interactions affecting behaviour, such as those moderated by complexly determined experiences, dispositions, abilities, attitudes, and affective states.

A simple way of formulating the conceptual shift here is that while plants are sessile—fixed or in motion only because of some outside force such as ocean currents—animals use their own energy resources to move, and individual animals can move to varying environments, up to the point of human beings who have multiple possibilities as to what kind of place to be in and what kind of thing to do—although this within the options available to us—this in turn altering environmental exposure. Insofar as individual differences play in selecting among possibilities, the outcomes will be attributable to the person's individual nature, though this in turn dependent on genes and prior exposures and learning. Life and lifestyle choices, within the options available to us, are themselves influenced by all the factors that make us what we are: genes, upbringing, learning, values.

This has the radical implication that genes can play a role in determining the environment as environmental exposures, in addition to the point above that environmental exposures can determine gene expression. In combination, the implication is that dynamic interplay is fundamental, not separate categories.

References

1. Varela, F. J., Thompson, E., & Rosch, E. (1991). *The embodied mind: Cognitive science and human experience.* Cambridge: The MIT Press.
2. Gillett, G. (2008). *Subjectivity and being somebody: Human identity and neuroethics.* Exeter: Imprint Academic.
3. Wilson, R.A., & Foglia, L. (2017). Embodied cognition. In E. N. Zalta (Ed.), *The stanford encyclopedia of philosophy* (Spring 2017 Edition), URL = https://plato.stanford.edu/archives/spr2017/entries/embodied-cognition/. Accessed 12/21/2018.
4. Newen, A., De Bruin, L., & Gallagher, S. (2018). *Oxford handbook of 4E cognition.* New York, NY: Oxford University Press.
5. Vygotsky, L. S. (1978). *Mind in society: The development of higher psychological processes.* Cambridge, MA: Harvard University Press.
6. Tollefsen, D., & Dale, R. (2018). Joint action and 4E cognition. In A. Newen, L. De Bruin, & S. Gallagher (Eds.), *The Oxford Handbook of 4E Cognition* (pp. 261–280). Oxford: Oxford University Press.
7. Merleau-ponty, M. (2012). *Phenomenology of Perception* (D. A. Landes, Trans.). New York: Routledge.
8. The science museum how does your brain work? http://www.sciencemuseum.org.uk/whoami/findoutmore/yourbrain/howdoesyourbrainwork/. Accessed October 7, 2017.
9. Descartes, R. (2003). *Discourse on method and meditations* (E. S. Haldane & G. R. T. Ross, Trans.). Mineola, New York: Dover Publications, Inc.
10. Aizawa, K., & Gillett, C. (2011). The autonomy of psychology in the age of neuroscience. In P. M. Illari, F. Russo, & J. Williamson (Eds.), *Causality in the sciences* (pp. 202–223). Oxford: Oxford University Press.
11. Bechtel, W. (2008). *Mental mechanisms: Philosophical perspectives on cognitive neuroscience.* London: Psychology Press.
12. The University of California. (2017). *Frontotemporal dementia.* http://memory.ucsf.edu/ftd/print/book/export/html/684. Accessed October 7, 2017.
13. Woodward, J. (2003). *Making things happen: A theory of causal explanation.* New York, NY: Oxford University Press.
14. Bolton, D. (1982). Life-form and idealism. *Royal Institute of Philosophy Lecture Series, 13,* 269–284.
15. Leckman, J. F., & March, J. S. (2011). Editorial: Developmental neuroscience comes of age. *Journal of Child Psychology and Psychiatry, 52*(4), 333–338. https://doi.org/10.1111/j.1469-7610.2011.02378.x.
16. Synofzik, M., Vosgerau, G., & Voss, M. (2013). The experience of agency: An interplay between prediction and postdiction. *Frontiers in Psychology, 4*(127). https://doi.org/10.3389/fpsyg.2013.00127.

17. Blakemore, S. J., & Choudhury, S. (2006). Development of the adolescent brain: Implications for executive function and social cognition. *Journal of Child Psychology and Psychiatry, 47*(3–4), 296–312. https://doi.org/10.1111/j.1469-7610.2006.01611.x.
18. Deci, E. L., & Ryan, R. M. (2000). The "what" and "why" of goal pursuits: Human needs and the self-determination of behavior. *Psychological Inquiry, 11*(4), 227–268. https://doi.org/10.1207/s15327965pli1104_01.
19. Bandura, A. (2006). Toward a psychology of human agency. *Perspectives on Psychological Science, 1*(2), 164–180. https://doi.org/10.1111/j.1745-6916.2006.00011.x.
20. Bandura, A. (2008). Reconstrual of "free will" from the agentic perspective of social cognitive theory. In J. Baer, J. C. Kaufman, & R. F. Baumeister (Eds.), *Are we free? Psychology and free will* (pp. 86–127). New York, NY: Oxford University Press.
21. Vygotsky, L. S. (1990). The genesis of higher mental functions. In K. Richardson & S. Sheldon (Eds.), *Cognitive development to adolescence* (pp. 61–80). Hove: Lawrence Erlbaum Associates.
22. Wittgenstein, L. (1953). *Philosophical Investigations* (G. E. M. Anscombe, Trans.). Oxford: Blackwell.
23. Eshleman, A. (2016). Moral responsibility. In E.N. Zalta (Ed.), *The stanford encyclopedia of philosophy* (Winter 2016 Edition). URL = <https://plato.stanford.edu/archives/win2016/entries/moral-responsibility/>. Accessed 12/21/2018.
24. Christman, J., & Anderson, N. (Eds.). (2005). *Autonomy and the challenges to liberalism.* Cambridge: Cambridge University Press.
25. Bolton, D., & Banner, N. (2012). Does mental disorder involve a loss of personal autonomy? In L. Radoilska (Ed.), *Autonomy and mental disorder* (pp. 77–99). Oxford: Oxford University Press.
26. Beauchamp, T. L., & Childress, J. F. (2012). *Principles of biomedical ethics* (7th ed.). New York, NY: Oxford University Press.
27. Marmot, M. (2006). Status syndrome: A challenge to medicine. *Journal of the American Medical Association, 295*(11), 1304–1307.
28. Hegel, G. W. (2009). *Phenomenology of Spirit*, (J. B. Baillie, Trans.). Lawrence, KS: Digireads.com. Original publication 1807.
29. Iser, M. (2013). Recognition. In E.N. Zalta (Ed.), *The stanford encyclopedia of philosophy* (Fall 2013 Edition), URL = <https://plato.stanford.edu/archives/fall2013/entries/recognition/>. Accessed 12/21/2018.
30. Taylor, C. (1992). The politics of recognition. In A. Gutmann (Ed.), *Multiculturalism: Examining the politics of recognition* (pp. 25–73). Princeton: Princeton University Press.
31. Williams, R. R. (1992). *Recognition: Fichte and Hegel on the other.* Albany, NY: SUNY Press.

32. Lasswell, H. (1936). *Politics: Who gets what, when, how.* New York: Whittlesey House.
33. Mackenzie, C., & Stoljar, N. (Eds.). (2000). *Relational autonomy: Feminist perspectives on autonomy, agency and the social self.* New York: Oxford University Press.
34. Delgado, R., & Stefancic, J. (2017). *Critical race theory* (3rd ed.). New York: New York University Press.
35. Loomba, A. (2015). *Colonialism/Postcolonialism* (3rd ed.). London: Routledge.
36. Fricker, M. (2007). *Epistemic injustice: Power and the ethics of knowing.* Oxford: Oxford University Press.
37. Dotson, K. (2011). Tracking epistemic violence, tracking practices of silencing. *Hypatia, 26*(2), 236–257. https://doi.org/10.1111/j.1527-2001.2011.01177.x.
38. Cockerham, W. C. (2007). *Social causes of health and disease.* Cambridge: Polity Press.
39. Kelly, M. P., Kelly, R. S., & Russo, F. (2014). The integration of social, behavioral, and biological mechanisms in models of pathogenesis. *Perspectives in Biology and Medicine, 57*(3), 308–328.
40. Krieger, N. (1994). Epidemiology and the web of causation: Has anyone seen the spider? *Social Science and Medicine, 39*(7), 887–903.
41. Krieger, N. (2008). Proximal, distal, and the politics of causation: What's level got to do with it? *American Journal of Public Health, 98*(2), 221–230.
42. Marmot, M. (2005). Remediable or preventable social factors in the aetiology and prognosis of medical disorders. In P. D. White (Ed.), *Biopsychosocial Medicine: An integrated approach to understanding illness* (pp. 39–58). New York: Oxford University Press.
43. Galea, S., Riddle, M., & Kaplan, G. A. (2010). Causal thinking and complex system approaches in epidemiology. *International Journal of Epidemiology, 39*(1), 97–106. https://doi.org/10.1093/ije/dyp296.
44. Heath, J. (2015). Methodological individualism. In E.N. Zalta (Ed.), *The stanford encyclopedia of philosophy* (Spring 2015 Edition), URL = <https://plato.stanford.edu/archives/spr2015/entries/methodological-individualism/>. Accessed 12/21/2018.
45. Zahle, J. (2016). Methodological holism in the social sciences. In E.N. Zalta (Ed.), *The stanford encyclopedia of philosophy* (Summer 2016 Edition), URL = <https://plato.stanford.edu/archives/sum2016/entries/holism-social/>. Accessed 12/21/2018.
46. List, C., & Spiekermann, K. (2013). Methodological individualism and holism in political science: A reconciliation. *American Political Science Review, 107*(4), 629–643. https://doi.org/10.1017/S0003055413000373.

47. UK Research Councils. (2017). *Widening cross-disciplinary research for mental health.* http://www.rcuk.ac.uk/documents/documents/cross-disciplinary-mental-health-research-agenda-pdf/. Accessed December 21, 2018.
48. Moffitt, T. E., Caspi, A., & Rutter, M. (2005). Strategy for investigating interactions between measured genes and measured environments. *Archives of General Psychiatry, 62*(5), 473–481. https://doi.org/10.1001/archpsyc.62.5.473.
49. Purcell, S. (2002). Variance components models for gene-environment interaction in twin analysis. *Twin Res, 5*(6), 554–571. https://doi.org/10.1375/136905202762342026.
50. Atkinson, N. J., & Urwin, P. E. (2012). The interaction of plant biotic and abiotic stresses: From genes to the field. *Journal of Experimental Botany, 63*(10), 3523–3543.
51. Weaver, I. C. G., Cervoni, N., Champagne, F. A., D'Alessio, A. C., Sharma, S., Seckl, J. R., et al. (2004). Epigenetic programming by maternal behavior. *Nature Neuroscience, 7*, 847. https://doi.org/10.1038/nn1276.
52. Robinson, G. E., Fernald, R. D., & Clayton, D. F. (2008). Genes and social behavior. *Science, 322*(5903), 896–900.
53. Anacker, C., O'Donnell, K. J., & Meaney, M. J. (2014). Early life adversity and the epigenetic programming of hypothalamic-pituitary-adrenal function. *Dialogues in Clinical Neuroscience, 16*(3), 321–333.
54. Talmud, P. J. (2007). Gene–environment interaction and its impact on coronary heart disease risk. *Nutrition, Metabolism and Cardiovascular Diseases, 17*(2), 148–152.
55. McGuinness, D., McGlynn, L. M., Johnson, P. C., MacIntyre, A., Batty, G. D., Burns, H., et al. (2012). Socio-economic status is associated with epigenetic differences in the pSoBid cohort. *International Journal of Epidemiology, 41*(1), 151–160. https://doi.org/10.1093/ije/dyr215.
56. Manuck, S. B., & McCaffery, J. M. (2014). Gene-environment interaction. *Annual Review of Psychology, 65*, 41–70.

CHAPTER 4

Biopsychosocial Conditions of Health and Disease

Abstract This chapter continues from the previous chapter on themes in biopsychosocial conditions of health and disease, picking up some core questions familiar in the theory and philosophy of medicine. We argue that the concepts and boundaries of health and disease are themselves biopsychosocial. Controversies about whether such-and-such a condition is or is not a medical matter, as opposed to difference or lifestyle choice, the consequences of being which involve benefits such as access to healthcare and/or harms such as stigma, and the terms in which such debates are conducted—are all thoroughly biopsychosocial-political. Core defining features of illness—activity limitations, pain and distress—likewise involve our psychology and social life as well as our biology. On the theme of causation, we endorse scientific method as the route to identifying causal mechanisms, note the major role of chronic stress in models of causal mechanisms linking psychosocial factors with biological damage, and spell out that chronic stress is a quintessential biopsychosocial concept. We consider the Research Domain Criteria (RDoC) proposed recently by the N.I.M.H. as a framework for research in mental health as an illustration of a biopsychosocial research framework, potentially extendable to cover physical health and biomedicine. Physical and mental health conditions are brought together in the new biopsychosocial model rather than being axiomatically separate—as they were in the old context of reductionism and dualism.

D. Bolton and G. Gillett,
The Biopsychosocial Model of Health and Disease,
https://doi.org/10.1007/978-3-030-11899-0_4

Keywords Biopsychosocial research framework · Causal mechanisms · Patient-centred care model · Recovery model · Pain · Social disability model · Research Domains Criteria (RDoC)

4.1 Conditions of Biopsychosocial Life

So far, we have reviewed the rationale as well as the challenges for the biopsychosocial model, in Chapter 1, and, drawing on contemporary life and human sciences, presented conceptualisations of the biological, in Chapter 2, and the psychological and social, in Chapter 3. In the later parts of Chapter 3, we drew out features of the biopsychosocial whole, especially that causal interactions run within and between these three, or rather four, since the natural environment is thoroughly involved with all, a point made explicit in Sect. 2.3. Critical for the biopsychosocial model as a model of health and disease, foundational biopsychosocial concepts already have the relevant normative distinction built into them. Chapter 2 characterised biological processes as local areas running contrary to the general direction of the second law of thermodynamics, temporarily; this feat achieved by metabolic regulatory mechanisms, which, as and when they fail, jeopardise the viability of the organism, which in any case eventually inevitably ends up back as dust, more or less prematurely. Some familiar conditions of biological life were listed in Sect. 3.3, such as food, water, oxygen, suitable ambient temperature, accommodation, on the way to the less obvious conditions of psychological life as agency, which include opportunity, access to resources such as education and training, which involves, picking up themes in Sect. 3.2, recognition by a supportive, encouraging and resourced social group, which is also necessary, along with peace and an uncompromised natural environment, for basic biological security.

In short, the conditions of biological, psychological and social life—risks and protective factors for developing and recovering from health conditions—are pervasive. As this has become clear in science and our thinking, health policy has recognised that it should be cross-sectoral, involving much more than the healthcare sector. As a general rule, the healthcare sector is trained and funded to treat people who have fallen below the or their normal level of functioning, in important domains, with the aim of restoration of function, or optimising lowered function, or reducing avoidable further loss. The healthcare sector also has a limited role in primary prevention, but this has turned out to be a multifaceted, cross-sectoral task, in which the illness-related language of healthcare gives way to more general concepts such as promoting resilience, or well-being, thriving, or further away still, happy enough family life, access to and use of educational opportunity, satisfying and well enough paid work, friendships and meaningful civic engagement.

The biopsychosocial model is a model of health and disease, but this roughly divides up, for reasons understandable in terms of the model, into, on the one hand, the business of the healthcare sector—illness, with the negative conception of health as avoidance of or recovery from illness—and, on the other hand, prevention of illness, which merges into resilience and thriving, which are protections against ill health from the point of view of healthcare, but which from all other, non-illness preoccupied sectors, are another thing altogether: education, work, economics, politics, environmental policy and security. In this fourth chapter, we pursue further implications of biopsychosocial theory as a model of disease and health as absence of disease, leaving aside the broader questions of health and well-being.

4.2 Biopsychosocial Conceptualisation of Health Conditions

Concepts and Boundary Disputes

Some questions about illness are causal and some conceptual, though there is no hard and fast line between them. Causal questions are about identifying risks, pathways and mechanisms of disease, developing clinical therapeutics and treatment technologies. They are questions for the basic and clinical sciences, and they take for granted what is disease and what is not. Or rather, to make clearer the conceptual point, the sciences are independent of whether the conditions of interest are called 'disease', and who by, as opposed to, for example, just phenotypic 'difference' or 'life-style choice', or 'sin'. These alternatives show up not much in science, but more in social, political, legal, moral and theological debate. They raise more or less far-reaching conceptual issues, to do with the meaning of 'illness', the logic of illness attribution and human nature. While scientific findings may be brought to bear on them, typically they cannot be settled by the science, or at least not to everyone's satisfaction, indicating that there are other relevant considerations. The main point of this section is that these conceptual questions are biopsychosocial. Here is Karl Jaspers on this point, in 1913 around the beginning of modern medicine and psychiatry, also noting that such questions do not normally merit medical attention [1] (p. 652):

> What health and illness mean in general are matters which concern the physician least of all. He deals scientifically with life processes and with particular illnesses. What is 'ill' in general depends less on the judgement of the doctor than on the judgment of the patient and on the dominant views in any given cultural circle.

In conditions of certainty, there is no need to spell out what *illness* means; all concerned, at home and in the hospital, know only too well, and they have other serious tasks to be getting on with. And if and when the need for a definition of *illness* or *disease* arises, in a textbook or classroom or the clinic, it is easy enough to give one simply by using some other term with similar meaning, such as *abnormal* structure or function, or *disruption*, *disturbance*, *dysregulation*, etc. The medical textbook descriptions of signs, syndromes and diseases are full of such terms, and they can all be used to define each other well enough for most purposes. This family of disease/illness related terms are all typically systemic, referring to abnormalities or disturbances of structural forms, regulation and functional ends.

The meaning of illness—and all the cognates to do with abnormality—becomes an issue in conditions of uncertainty and dispute as to whether such and such a condition is an illness or not, in circumstances when it seems that no further observation or laboratory test would settle the matter clearly one way or the other. This uncertainty arises when criteria that normally go together, in the paradigm or prototypical kind of case, fall apart. Three key features of illness typically go together: the person complains of distress or pain; second, they are unable to do things they need to do, there is incapacity or activity limitation, loss of agency; and third, there is the assumption that these things are because something is not well with the person's body or mind. This last assumption implies that medical/psychological expertise is required, hopefully, to reduce the harm (the distress/pain and incapacity) and not create more. When these features and assumptions are all present and correct, there are conditions for certainty—but insofar as they cleave apart, some present, some absent, or dubious, the position becomes ambiguous; attribution of illness and the closely linked perceived need for healthcare professional attention, become uncertain. With uncertainty comes controversy. Examples of general kinds of case where attribution of illness and/or need for medical attention is commonly contested include: some mental health diagnoses, especially those associated with non-voluntary admissions; 'medically unexplained' conditions; alleged over-medicalising and overtreating of conditions that are regarded rather as 'normal', self-limiting, or less harmful compared with harms from treating; pathologising/stigmatising difference and diversity, and lifestyle choices—even if they carry raised risk of illness.

The reference to 'pathologizing/stigmatising'refers to a downside of the illness attribution—a harmful side effect, linked to the main effect. The main effect of illness is to decrease our agency, up to and including the ultimate ending of it all. The adverse effects of illness on agency, and the experience of illness as pain and distress, cue interpersonal and institutionalised responses to help, to provide resources including care and treatment. At the same time, social expectations are reduced: the ill person is excused from normal social role obligations, from moral responsibility, and hence from blame; the attribution of causation of behaviour, or of inactivity, is to the illness, not to the person as agent. In short, illness attribution implies excuse for and not being blamed for the downturn in functioning, and the right to access available healthcare. However, at the same time, and for the same reasons, pathologising carries the risk of disqualification of the person from their full recognition as a self-determining agent in the social world—with knock-on risks of being stigmatised and subjected to the many varieties of social exclusion. The relative benefits and losses of being seen as ill depend on many general and individual factors. For sudden onset, treatable conditions, the benefits are typically high and the costs (of the above psychosocial sort) relatively low. For long-term conditions, with no treatment, or with treatments that—from the person's point of view—may do as much harm as good, the balance shifts, costs may outweigh benefits, leading to a rejection of the 'illness' label, in favour of 'difference' and 'diversity'.

Conditions of so-called 'disability' are a special case, distinguished from 'illness', for complex reasons including absence of treatment, and, commonly, the absence of complaints of distress. However, the 'disability' label functions like the 'illness' label in that it imputes deficit in ability, hence excuse from 'normal' social role obligations, and hence at the same time carries risk of demotion from full recognition as an equal agent. Furthermore, for lifelong conditions, 'disability' is not relative to the person's own previous functioning, and for acquired chronic conditions, the downturn in personal functioning does not come with implied upturn, and becomes 'difference'. The implication is that the critical notion of 'deficit in relation to normal' is benchmarked not against the person's own normality but against normality of the majority. Further, since ability to act is a function not only of personal abilities but that always in the context of task demands and available resources and opportunities, the cause of 'disability' can be legitimately attributed to these external factors; for example, people who have to use wheelchairs are handicapped in mobility by the way the majority build transport systems, not by their condition in itself. These kinds of points are well theorised in the 'social model of disability' (e.g. [2, 3]).

In short, conceptual issues around illness—and disability-related concepts and practices involve a complex range of and interaction between biological, psychological, social, moral and policy factors. They cannot be so much as articulated without a full biopsychosocial framework.

The Logic of Disease Attribution Is Top-Down

The fundamental feature of disease in a system is that it causes—or significantly raises risk of—disruption of the function of the system, thus leading to adverse outcomes for a dependent system. 'Adverse outcomes for a dependent system' implies disruption of functionality of that dependent system, and that dysfunctionality in turn means that it causes or raises of adverse outcomes on a further dependent system… and so on. This cascade continues until we reach dysfunctionality/adverse outcomes for the organism as a whole in its activity in the environment. It is poor outcomes at the level of the whole that ultimately drives attribution of dysfunctionality downwards to the parts that serve the whole. In short, the difference between function and dysfunction (or between good enough function and not good enough function) of parts, ultimately turns on the difference between function and dysfunction (or between good enough function and not good enough function) of the organism as a whole.

In short, the logic of disease attribution is top-down, not bottom-up. The causal pathways, by contrast, can be bottom-up, as for example atherosclerosis causing an embolus causing cardiac arrest causing the person's death. Causal pathways can also be top-down as previously considered; for example, chronic unhealthy diet and lack of exercise raising risk for atherosclerosis. But the point made here is a different one, namely, that the logic of dysfunction, as opposed to function, is top-down, in the sense that it flows from whole to part.

The Centrality of the Person

The implication of the line of argument in the preceding section is that, in biopsychosocial systems theory, health conditions have to be understood in terms of the person as a whole, specifically how it affects their agency, values and achievement of personal goals. The centrality of the person was identified by Engel as a feature of the biopsychosocial model in his original papers [4, 5]. In this respect, there are some connections between the biopsychosocial model and the Patient- or Client-centred Care Model, and many papers have examined the relation between the two approaches (e.g. [6–9]).

There are also connections with the Recovery model, a relatively recent, important and radical influence on mental health services [10–12]. The model focuses on chronic health conditions, on the centrality of the person's life and values, on achieving a good quality-of-life, on the need for good medical and nursing care, especially in acute phases, and on issues of access to social resources and opportunities. Many if not all aspects of the Recovery model can be applied as much to chronic physical health conditions as to mental health conditions, though so far this extension is in its infancy (see e.g. [13]).

The focus on chronic conditions has implications for a distinction often drawn in the literature between *illness* and *disease*, illness being the condition of the person, and hence involved in the personal and social world, and disease being a dysfunctional condition of a bodily organ or system, and not so involved (e.g. [14, 15]). Although this is an important distinction, it applies most clearly in cases where there is an identifiable somatic disease process, in an otherwise unaffected person, which subsequently remits, spontaneously or with treatment. The distinction becomes blurred, however, in chronic conditions that have to be accommodated in the person's life and hence involved with the development of the whole personality. William Osler's famous remark: It is much more important to know what sort of a patient has a disease than what sort of a disease a patient has [16]—applies especially well to chronic conditions. This blurring of the difference between disease and illness is another aspect of the shift from the (infectious) disease paradigm to focus on non-communicable conditions, which require a biopsychosocial approach.

This shift affects the definitions of health and disease. A recent BMJ article by an international group [17] critiques the 1948 WHO definition of health as 'complete physical, mental and social well-being and not merely the absence of disease or infirmity'. The authors acknowledge the definition's groundbreaking breath and ambition at the time, going on to criticisms, mainly unintentional contribution to the medicalisation of society, continuing to the second problem, arising from the increasing relative prevalence of long-term conditions [17] (p. 1):

> The number of people living with chronic diseases for decades is increasing worldwide… In this context, the WHO definition becomes counterproductive as it declares people with chronic diseases and disabilities definitively ill. It minimises the role of the human capacity to cope autonomously with life's ever changing physical, emotional, and social challenges and to function with fulfilment and a feeling of wellbeing with a chronic disease or disability.

Consistent with this last sentence, the authors go on to propose a conceptualisation of health as the *ability to adapt and to self-manage*, discussing this in relation to physical health, mental health and social health.

A concept of health along these lines makes personal agency fundamental, though in its broad biopsychosocial context, interacting with resources and opportunities. A person's sense of agency, whether they can do enough to have a viable life, and with it whether they wish for life, as it is, or better, with treatment or with none, are all matters that depend on the person. The condition of the biological body matters, but insofar as it affects the person. It is of fundamental importance in healthcare that it is the person who feels ill and wants treatment, any or more, or feels well enough without it. We attend to the person, not the body part—and not to psychological signs and symptoms in isolation either. The centrality of the person also shows up in the next section. We will quote from Wittgenstein: the pain may be in the hand, but we comfort the person, not the hand.

Pain and Distress Have Personal Biopsychosocial Meaning

Activity limitation is the core behavioural feature of illness or injury, *pain* and *distress* are their subjectively experienced aspects. But even these subjective experiences turn out to be thoroughly biopsychosocial, whichever way one approaches them: by philosophical analysis of 'subjective experience', or in terms of neuropsychological models of causal pathways, or behavioural models of interpersonal pain signalling functions.

Cartesian dualism has had a massive impact on our folk way of thinking about subjective experience, especially inclination to suppose that it is essentially *separated from the body* and *private to the person*. One of the key philosophical critiques of what could be called 'folk dualism' (as opposed to the full-blown complex, original Cartesian metaphysics linked to the mechanisation of the world-picture) is by Ludwig Wittgenstein in his *Philosophical Investigations*, much of which anticipates the kind of philosophical framework we are proposing in this book. Here is a conclusion of Wittgenstein's discussion of the meaning of 'pain' [18] (para. 281):

> 'But doesn't what you say come to this: that there is no pain, for example, without *pain-behaviour?*' It comes to this: only of a living human being and what resembles (behaves like) a living human being can one say: it has sensations; it sees; is blind; hears; is deaf; is conscious or unconscious.

Expressed in the terms of 'dynamical forms', which we have used throughout in explicating biopsychosocial theory, it is the human living form that has psychology. This is a fundamental aspect of the non-dualist idea of 'embodiment', considered previously in Sect. 3.1. In the same movement of thought, Wittgenstein finds a simple way of making clear that the human being has a special 'centre'—the 'I', the person's speech and face—involved in recognition [18] (para. 286):

> But isn't it absurd to say of a *body* that it has pain?——And why does one feel an absurdity in that? In what sense is it true that my hand does not feel pain, but I in my hand? What sort of issue is: Is it the *body* that feels pain?—How is it to be decided? What makes it plausible to say that it is *not* the body?— Well, something like this: if someone has a pain in his hand, then the hand does not say so (unless it writes it) and one does not comfort the hand, but the sufferer: one looks into his face.

Reconstructions of pain that involve moving away from preconceptions of mind/body dualism, appear increasingly in the humanities literatures (e.g. [19, 20]).

Turning to the science of pain, this is an expanding, large and complex area of research and we give a very brief and simplified survey of some relevant key points. Until about the mid-1960s, it was supposed that pain was caused by signalling of tissue damage to the central nervous system by specific pathways. In the 1960s, Ronald Melzack and Patrick Wall [21] proposed their innovative 'gate theory' to supersede specificity models, explaining how pain perception involved multiple neural pathways, creating a model more able to capture individual and cultural contextual factors in pain perception. Melzack and Wall's theory created the foundations for increasingly sophisticated models of pain perception, involving both bottom-up and central, context-sensitive pathways. In a chapter on the subject the neuroscientist Howard Fields describes current models of neurological pathways of pain perception and then considers its signalling functions—its meaning for the person, using the example of inadvertently touching a hot iron [22] (pp. 44–45):

> Turning to the subjective experience: there are three distinct components [...] First, there is the purely discriminative part that includes recognizing the quality of the sensation as a burn and localizing it to your hand. Second, there is the motivational aspect associated with the desire to pull your hand away or to terminate the sensation. Third, there is an evaluative component *the thought of the damage that has been done to your hand and how that will affect your life in the hours and days ahead.* (italics added)

It is this third component—italicised in the quotation above—that is of special interest here, because we take it to involve: the thought of the impact of the damage to oneself, one's agency and way of life, including its always important social aspects. In short, this evaluative component that is central to the experience of pain is thoroughly biopsychosocial. The 'biopsychosocial' appears here in the *intentionality* of pain, i.e. in what it is 'about', its meaning or representational content, which is, briefly: threat of loss of significant biopsychosocial function.

These considerations also provide a way of comparing 'physical pain' with 'psychological pain', or 'distress'. As a simplification, psychological pain or distress is high on negative thoughts and feelings about one's prospects. Fields has this [22] (p. 46):

> In addition to its role in pain perception, the limbic system mediates emotional responses to a variety of factors including personal loss, anticipation of harm, and so on. The dysphoric states such as depression and anxiety share limbic system circuits with somatic pain. It is thus no accident that the word "pain" is often used to denote emotional pain that has no somatic component.

The evaluative component in pain perception figures prominently in psychological models of pain and distress, with clinical applications. Highly negative (fearful) appraisals about the effect of damage, or other negative events, and indeed of the pain or distress itself, on one's future life are sometimes referred to as *catastrophizing*, and they typically risk having the effect of amplifying the experience. These models have the implication that psychological management of pain and distress should target among other things reduction of catastrophising [23].

A further psychosocial aspect of pain and distress is their function in interpersonal signalling and regulation of behaviour. This aspect is already implied in Wittgenstein's account of pain expression: expressions of pain, behavioural, facial and verbal, induce caring responses from others. It has been theorised in various ways, for example in the Social Communication Model of Pain [24] and in evolutionary theoretic terms [25].

4.3 Locating Causes in Biopsychosocial Systems

Identifying Dysfunctions and Modifiable Causes

While disease is contextualised in the person as a whole, the immediate question is where the dysfunctional process is located: which system within the whole is dysfunctional, causing problems for the whole? The methodological assumption of healthcare is that the person as a whole is in trouble because of some dysfunctional part, a dysfunctional subsystem within the body/mind. It underlies the traditional individual focussed medical model of identification of clinical syndromes and diagnoses, and models of psychological processes in the individual that give rise to distress and activity limitations. The scientific details are in the medical and clinical psychological textbooks and will not be taken further here. We focus more on the broader implications of systems theory and the biopsychosocial approach. The main issue is that systems theory envisages (causal) interactions everywhere, including within and between the organism and the environment, in which context the question arises: what is the logic of attributing causes of dysfunction to the organism rather than the environment?

In systems theory, one cannot begin to talk about the function of systems without reference to their operating environments. All biological systems function in interaction with others and ultimately in relation to fitness of the whole organism in a range of environmental conditions. One broad kind of pathway to dysfunction of the whole is poorness of fit between the expected environment, to which behaviour is adapted, and the actual environment, to which it isn't. This general point applies in the evolutionary context, for example in the so-called 'thrifty phenotype' hypothesis applied to obesity. Hales and Barker [26] hypothesise that in poor dietary conditions in utero metabolic mechanisms are set to maximise fat storage in expectation of subsequent, poor post-natal dietary intake; this mechanism would be highly adaptive in environments where poor dietary conditions in utero were reliably followed by poor dietary conditions postnatal, as may be reasonably assumed to be the case in our original evolutionary environments; but if this association breaks down, as in postnatal dietary environments that are actually high in accessible sugar/fats, the consequence would be a hard to modify tendency to excessive fat storage. The general idea of poorness of fit of previously adaptive mechanisms to later environments has an ontogenetic version in the learning theories in psychological science: behaviour shaped up by one set of environmental contingencies may be maladaptive in a subsequent environment. For example, if toddlers are reared in parenting styles involving multiple and conflicting commands, the child is likely to learn to ignore them and to seek to satisfy their own goals regardless, but this behaviour pattern will likely lead to poor outcomes in the classroom [27, 28].

Notwithstanding these considerations, we still locate the problem—the dysfunction—in the person. An obvious reason for doing so is the centrality of the person: it is the person to whom harm accrues—who suffers pain, distress, significant impairment of agency and loss. However, this consideration alone is superficial in a systemic context, because the cause may still lie outside the person, being done to, and this is the force behind the social model of disability which we have already had occasion to cite in this section. A more promising key to this issue is the one increasingly found in the health literature: the concept of identifying modifiable causes. The idea is that, among all the criss-crossing causal pathways, what needs to be identified are promising targets for intervention. This approach is consistent with the interventionist approach to causality referred to in Chapter 3, Sect. 3.1, and is well suited to healthcare as applied science, seeking to change things, for the better. From this point of view, dysfunction attribution is in part—and somewhat paradoxically—shorthand for belief about promising possibilities for change. While 'dysfunction' and its cognates connote deficit, promising possibilities for change are opportunities.

In complex systems where there is a poor fit between the person's behaviours and the environment, the question arises: where is potential for change? In conditions of the person that are lifelong, not amenable to change, the potential for change lies elsewhere, not in the person, but in social attitudes and resources—and this is a compelling argument of the social model of disability. For acquired long-term health conditions, it is likely that optimal outcomes from the person's point of view come from a combination of—in no order—available high-quality healthcare, self-management, social support, plus non-discrimination by broader society.

Effective treatment or prevention technologies rely on targeting a cause of large enough effect, i.e. a causal factor identified in group studies that accounts for a large proportion of the outcome variance. The main point for the present purpose is that there are few causes of currently common health conditions with so large an effect that targeting them leads to complete prevention or complete cure, and for the majority, a multimodal approach to multiple factors is required.

These issues relate to the problem of *reduction of disease to a single primary cause*. If a normal function of a biological system is carried out by only that one system, then the failure of that function will be reducible to processes within that one system. For example, insofar as it is only the cardiovascular system that delivers oxygen to cells, failure to achieve that functional end, depleted oxygen delivery to cells, is attributable only to—and in this sense is reducible to—cardiovascular dysfunction, to a cardiovascular disease process such as atherosclerosis. In many cases however, and this may be the general rule, biological functions are affected by multiple subsystems, with the effect that achievement of a particular function is not a matter of processes in any one system, but may be affected by many interacting systems. However, such factors may not be relevant to the disease process once onset: for example, advanced arteriosclerosis is not likely to be reversed by social policy affecting dietary changes, and quite different interventions may be needed, such as bypass surgery. On the other hand, for acquired, chronic health conditions, there is typically ongoing interaction with environmental, psychological and social factors. There is, in brief, no reduction to a primary cause, biological, psychological or social, but rather multiple systems of all kinds are involved at varying stages, some contributing risk for poor outcomes, others contributing to protection, including restorative and compensatory mechanisms.

Identifying Causal Mechanisms

In setting the scene for developing biopsychosocial theory in the first chapter, we noted that evidence of biological, psychological and social causal factors in many health conditions comes from group statistical data in controlled study designs. The inference to causation relies on the empiricist approach to causation, after Hume and Mill, as association or correlation determined in experimental or quasi-experimental study designs. We noted however that such data in themselves provide no theoretical account of what kind of thing the variables stand for, or what kind of causal properties they have, separately or in combination. This absence of ontological-causal theory is particularly noticeable given the long-standing assumptions that physical(-chemical) processes alone are causal, covered by inviolable physical laws, that therefore biological factors can be causal only because biology is physics and chemistry, while mental events are scientifically odd epiphenomena, and social processes can hardly be conceptualised at all within this particular world view. The task of Chapter 3 and this chapter is to elucidate a general biopsychosocial theory capable of comprehending biopsychosocial data.

Issues raised by untheorised statistical data appear in the philosophy of medicine literature in discussion of whether the empiricist approach to determining causes, using controlled study designs and associated statistical methods, is sufficient, or whether it is also necessary to identify *causal mechanisms*. Federica Russo and Jon Williamson have proposed [29] (p. 158):

> The health sciences infer causal relations from mixed evidence: on the one hand, mechanisms and theoretical knowledge, and, on the other, statistics

> and probabilities. Statistics are used to show that the cause makes a difference to the effect, and mechanisms allow causal relationships to explain the occurrence of an effect.

This proposal turns on what a 'causal mechanism' is, and specifically on whether identifying a causal mechanism is distinct from determining probabilities in controlled study designs. In their paper cited above Russo and Williamson give examples of causal mechanisms, and in a related paper, Illari and Williamson [30] (p. 1) cite a definition of 'causal mechanism' from Machamer et al. [31]: 'entities and activities organized in such a way that they are responsible for the phenomenon'—which is somewhat vague with more than a hint of circularity. A more informative definition is provided by Glennan [32] (S 344):

> A mechanism for a behaviour is a complex system that produces that behaviour by the interaction of a number of parts, where the interactions between parts can be characterised by direct, invariant, change relating generalisations.

This is more informative, but is so exactly because it reintroduces the importance of invariant generalisations consistent with the empiricist approach to causation.

So what is a causal mechanism over and over what is established by controlled experimentation? The life sciences deal with complex systems changing over time, with probabilistic associations between inputs and outputs that are separated spatially by the inner workings of the system and by time. Confidence in having identified a causal mechanism is raised when the events are proximate, with fewer or no intervening processes and closer in time. So one idea behind 'causal mechanism' is just that we *fill in the intervening steps*, spatial and temporal, finding causal connections of ever closer proximity between inputs and effects, between, for example, environmental exposures at one time and poor health at a later time. This approach to 'causal mechanism'—filling in the intermediate steps—is suggested by Illari and Williamson [30], and supported by considerations in, for example, Kincaid [33]. It is, however, readily accommodated in the empiricist approach to causation, a point well-argued by Kendler and Campbell [34]. A corollary of filling in the intervening steps, with ever closer proximity of links in the causal chain, taking into account other proximate factors at each step, in effect increases probabilities from lower to higher. Further, as probabilities of association and correlations approach 1, the sample size required for confidence in generalisability reduces: a few well-designed, replicated experiments with relatively small samples will do. All this can be understood in terms of the empiricist approach.

There is however the famous limitation of empiricist epistemology, whether in the knowledge of causes or knowledge generally, namely, that it omits *theory*, envisaging knowledge by observation only. In the statement of their thesis quoted above Russo and Williamson bring together '(causal) mechanisms and theoretical knowledge' contrasted with statistics and probabilities, but it is worth distinguishing them. It is true that experimental method or approximations to it only ever establish correlations and associations, albeit generalisable and counter-factual that can support intervention to make a difference. The theory goes further, however, explaining why the correlations exist and why the intervention works, 'explaining' in the sense of fitting into a more or less well-established body of knowledge. On the other hand, it should be said that the additional need for theory is not a totally different requirement compared with establishing causal connections; rather, theory is typically a broader class of causal connections, themselves established or confirmed using experimental methodologies or approximations. So, if we elucidate the concept of 'causal mechanism' in terms of 'theory', just as if we elucidate it in terms of intervening steps, the process of identifying a causal mechanism and identifying a cause are similar—and specifically, identifying causal mechanisms is not a separate epistemological route to establishing causes. This conclusion is consistent with Alex Broadbent's discussion of these issues in epidemiology [35], and with Bert Leuridan's and Erik Weber's discussion of mechanistic evidence and the International Agency for Research on Cancer (IARC) [36].

As to what theorised biopsychosocial causal mechanisms are, the general concepts and principles have been the main topic in preceding chapters, including *systems*, *structures* or *forms*, *functioning towards ends*, *information and communication*, *coding*, *regulation* and *control*. And for causal mechanisms responsible for breakdown, their relevant negations, such as such as *error*, *abnormal*, *dysfunction* and *dysregulation*. These are the general concepts and principles; the specifics are diverse, depending on which system, vulnerable structures, ends and control mechanisms are being modelled.

Stress as a Biopsychosocial Causal Mechanism

One of the most theorised and researched general causal mechanism for explaining biopsychosocial impacts on health is *stress*. Chronic stress, specifically, is hypothesised to be a key mechanism leading to stress-related biological reactivity such as inflammatory responses that adversely affect the immune system and other organs, raising the risk for a range of health conditions [37–40]. As an example of recent work in this area, here are summary statements from a recent major longitudinal study in *The Lancet* on the relation between resting amygdalar activity and cardiovascular events [41] (p. 2):

> Chronic stress carries an attributable risk for cardiovascular disease that is on par with other recognised risk factors, such as smoking, increased lipid concentrations, hypertension, and diabetes. Despite the prevalence and potency of this risk factor, little is known about the mechanisms that translate stress into cardiovascular disease events… Our study provides several observations that together define a mechanism linking stress to cardiovascular events…, specifically that the amygdala could be a key structure in the mechanism… and that upregulation of haemopoietic tissue activity and increased atherosclerotic inflammation are additionally implicated in a neural–haemopoietic–arterial axis.

In the experimental psychology literature spanning animal and human research, the concept of stress is closely linked to fear, anxiety and depression. Stress ors are various kinds of (perceived) threat, but with the specific feature of (perceived) *uncontrollability*. This idea has a long history in learning and personality psychology, for example, in Rotter's locus of control theory [42] and Seligman's learned helplessness model of depression [43]. Here is a formulation by Richard Lazarus [44] (p. 58):

> A good way of thinking about stressful person-environment relationships is to examine the relative balance of forces between environmental demands and the person's psychological resources for dealing with them. If the environmental load substantially exceeds the person's resources, a stressful relationship exists… In psychological stress, the comparison is between the power of the environmental demands to harm, threaten, or challenge, and the psychological resources of the person to manage these demands… From the standpoint of this way of thinking, stress is particularly powerful

> when the individual must struggle with demands that cannot easily be met… If the ratio of demands to resources becomes too great, we are no longer talking about high stress but trauma… The person feels helpless to deal with the demands to which he or she is exposed, and this can result in feelings of panic, hopelessness, and depression.

Psychologically, stress arises from exposure to salient negative, uncontrollable events, jeopardising the sense of agency. Salience covers what is essential to our biological and psychological life. Further, psychological stress essentially involves social factors such as task demands and access to resources. At the same time psychological stress is also biological, physiological: it is the activation of the arousal system, preparing for action to achieve important goals—but if the goals cannot be achieved, ever, or never enough, or never reliably, the arousal system is chronically active, and it is this chronic (hyper-) activity of the arousal system that is hypothesised to be the source of long-term biological damage. In short, chronic stress as the key hypothesised mechanism linking psychosocial factors with poor physical and mental health outcomes is—as to be expected—a mechanism that explicitly addresses criss-crossing biological, psychological and social processes. Key features of the hypothesised chronic stress mechanism are aspects of the core features we have proposed for biopsychosocial theory: the psychological sense of agency and action itself are compromised, raising risk for mental health problems, because social task demands are excessive and social resources inadequate, and the consequences of this chronic psychosocial misfortune is top-down dysregulation of critical biological processes raising risk of physical health problems.

Biopsychosocial Research Framework

The biopsychosocial model, like the narrower biomedical model, is not a scientific theory or summary of scientific findings, but could be applied as a framework for organising and planning research. The N.I.M.H. Research Domains Criteria RDoC framework for mental health is a rigorously worked out example of a framework in this sense [45]. The RDoC framework is a 2-dimensional grid: the columns are for biological, psychological and social factors—in this sense, the RDoC framework is explicitly biopsychosocial—and the rows refer to specific neural-psychological-behavioural systems (such as *fear* and *reward* systems). The cells can accommodate what is assumed known with more or less confidence, or could indicate what remains unknown, either not yet investigated or with mixed or inconclusive findings. We consider the RDoC research framework here because it is the best current and because it could be elaborated in various ways to have broader scope appropriate for the biopsychosocial model, for example application to physical health as well as mental health, incorporating biomedicine, and inclusion of a wider range and number of factors known to effect health and disease at various stages. Here are some main points that would be involved in such an elaboration:

- *Extension to physical health*: A research framework of this sort could be to apply to biological systems below as well as above the neck, to include such as the cardiovascular system as well as the central nervous system, in effect incorporating biomedicine, and potentially then able to have relevance to physical as well as to mental health conditions. Importantly, it would be able to accommodate the many kinds of pathways and conditions that do not fit neatly into either of these two categories, such as risks involving chronic stress, or the so-called psychosomatic conditions or medically unexplained symptoms. The expanded framework would in effect have the advantage of recognising interactions between the brain and other biological systems, and hence be able to accommodate the emerging evidence outlined in Chapter 1, Sect. 1.2, implicating psychosocial factors in the aetiology and course of medical conditions. Assuming the grid has explicit relevance to both systemic function and dysfunction in the rows, on which more below, some aspects of research findings relevant on mental health on the one hand and physical health on the other would diverge significantly, for example, confirmation of primary biological progressive disease mechanisms and treatments in some physical diseases. But in other areas of the grid, particularly relating to aetiological risk factors accumulating through the lifespan, or in areas of the grid—to be proposed for addition below—on management of chronic conditions and factors affecting quality-of-life, similarities among mental and physical health conditions would be more apparent.
- *More discrimination among kinds of psychological and social factors relevant to health and disease.* For example, to accommodate aspects of agency: agency as perceived, and agency related to social

factors including task demands (e.g. work; dependents) and access to resources and opportunities (these of many kinds, including access to treatment). This would require more columns. The RDoC framework is work in progress, adaptable as the science develops; current versions have around 5 columns for biological factors, around 1 for psychological, and around 0–1 for social factors (e.g. [45, 46]).

- *Acknowledgment of non-social environmental health risks*, especially important if physical health is included, again requiring more columns, to include factors such as ambient air quality and available diet.
- *Explicit specification of health conditions or 'diseases'*, not only the biological systems. The RDoC framework at present has no explicit conceptualisation or characterisation of mental health conditions, connected with the aim of replacing current psychosocial diagnostic criteria with biological criteria [47–49]. To accommodate specification of health conditions, probably a third dimension of the grid would be needed. This is easier to see if we imagine the grid incorporating biomedicine in which the issues are better worked out: the rows would be specific systems such as the immune system, with implicit reference to its components and functions, and the columns would specify factors affecting functioning, but probably a third dimension of the grid, distinct though theoretically closely connected to the rows and the columns, would be needed to specify the dysfunctions and disorders of the immune system. The cells in this now 3-dimensional grid could then accommodate findings of the specific subsystems responsible for harmful health conditions warranting healthcare attention.
- *Need to discriminate among stages of health conditions* would arise once a dimension specifically for health conditions was explicitly in place. It would also be necessary, as we have emphasised previously, to distinguish between research questions referring to, first, aetiology of disease incidence, in population samples; second, disease progression or maintenance, in patient samples; and third, factors affecting quality-of-life in chronic conditions. These discriminations are necessary because they are distinct research questions, requiring distinctive methodologies and sampling, and also—especially relevant to our main theme—because the balance of biological, psychological and social involvement can vary substantially depending

on the stage of a condition. For example, for cardiovascular disease biological processes dominate as maintaining factors and targets for intervention such as surgery in the advanced stages of the disease; whereas, if the question is the aetiology of cardiovascular disease, accumulation of risk factors in the population, to be applied as basis for prevention technologies, or application to advising an at-risk individual patient, then lifestyle social and factors, such as exercise and time of access to treatment, figure large. And for chronic diseases, in fact for all diseases where the person is alive and managing, not in coma, there are always issues of agency and the quality of life. A framework for organising or planning research into management of chronic diseases would, therefore, need to accommodate the full range of biological, psychological, environmental and social factors.

- *Population level as opposed to individual level questions*, for example, incidence vs. susceptibility, might require different grids, the one to do with differences between individuals (types), the other differences between populations. The UK NICE conceptual framework for public health [50], for example, distinguishes between individual and population patterns of disease and their causal mechanisms; both include biological, social and related factors, but the latter has additional interactions with a range of other factors including political and economic.
- Finally, a further dimension of variation is *developmental*. All biological and psychological systems in health and disease have developmental trajectories, within which there is variation in the relative influence of biopsychosocial and environmental factors, including in factors affecting vulnerability and resilience to adversities and illness. Hence all the research questions would have to allow for age variation.

The points above indicate what, based on considerations so far in this essay, would constitute an adequate framework for organising health research and identifying areas of relatively certainty and important unknowns. Possibly further dimensions could be added, for example on 'impact', estimating the relative importance of knowing more about a specific health condition at a specific stage, for treatment or prevention, depending on, for example, prevalence, projected prevalence, among what age-group, healthcare costs, associated cross-sectoral costs, etc. But, in any case, the elaborated framework as sketched above is already multidimensional, needs far more than a two-dimensional grid, can hardly be represented diagrammatically, though could be split up into different diagrams, but it is bound to be complicated if able to accommodate and organise the entire basic and clinical science health research—this can hardly be expected to be simple. In practice of course such a multidimensional monster grid to organise biopsychosocial research across the whole of healthcare will never be constructed because too big, too complicated and of no practical use. Small segments of the hypothetical framework are written up in reviews for circumscribed specifics: for some conditions, some treatments, some stages, some health economic analyses, some policies, other angles. Otherwise, it exists in the scientific literature as a whole, broadly construed, across the range of biopsychosocial and environmental sciences applied to health.

In the next section, we consider the tension—intrinsic to healthcare as it has developed over the past few decades—between research data of the kinds considered above, on groups, and clinical care of the individual.

Clinical Epistemology

It is something of an irony that while health research has made such strides over the past few decades, while knowledge has increased, certainty in the clinic is just as likely to have gone down as up! This is connected with the fact that much of what has been discovered is about complex, multifactorial causation. We know more about the body and mind, their functions and dysfunctions, and their interaction with the environment, and more about the treatment of biological and psychological health problems, but this has come along with increasing appreciation of the complexity of the problems, beyond physically damaged tissue or biological infection, involving multiple interacting biological systems, along with increased understanding of regulating systems with wide interactive reach, including the central nervous system and psychological functioning. Linked with multifactorial complexity, this new complicated knowledge is statistical, based on group studies, delivering associations such as relative risk and odds ratios, and quantifications of treatment effects such as effect size and number-needed-to-treat—and how all these statistics relate to a particular patient is unsettled. Notwithstanding the benefits of evidence-based practice, the challenges of inference from population-based aetiological risk studies and clinical treatment trials to preventative management and treatment of the individual patient are significant [51, 52]. The challenges here do not disqualify the application of the experimental method, following Mill's methods of agreement and difference, or approximations to them, to determine causes and effects (as outlined in Chapter 1, Sect. 1.3, under the heading "Biopsychosocial Data in Search of Theory"). There are in fact no other serious players on this particular pitch. Application includes reliance on randomised controlled treatment trials (or better, meta-analyses of multiple such trials) as being the most logically valid way of identifying treatment effects (see e.g. [53]). Experimental method can result in reliable positive findings, but also, and of high importance, reliable negative findings, likelihoods of no or no clinically significant effect of a treatment, compared with no treatment, or with a harmless placebo. The epistemological problem is not how to establish that a treatment technology has some effect or no effect in group samples, but rather that, because of many kinds of complexity (in the condition, in the sampling, in individual differences), treatments are rarely effective for all individuals, and application of the data to care of the individual patient is not straightforward. For this, as is often said, thorough assessment and clinical judgement are needed to combine with knowledge of the basic and clinical science.

Complexity and uncertainty are most marked where there is evidence of causation by multiple factors of small effect. Conversely, simplicity and certainty are most marked where single, primary causative factors are presumed. The single, primary factor approach works well in some specialist areas of biomedicine and psychological therapy, and less well in clinical settings with caseload is not restricted to a narrow range of conditions, in settings such as primary care, palliative care, care of the elderly, and community mental health. Other limitations of the single factor approach are apparent in medical wards and outpatient clinics in which some patients present with pain, distress and activity limitations in the absence of biomedically determined conditions. All these contexts require a broader causal theory, more complex, about which much is unknown at present, to do with biological/psychological/social interactions of the sort being explored for example in the chronic pain, health psychology and public health literatures.

This new complexity creates much uncertainty, in clinicians, patients and students. It can be resolved by a dogmatic certainty that the real cause must be one or another sort—something biological, psychological or social—though at the cost of selective inattention to other factors, the risk of over-reliance on one treatment approach, and detachment from anomalies. More adaptively, the uncertainty has to be tolerated. The more responsibility a clinician has, the more obligation they have to know the science as well as the patient and to keep a mind open to complexity and alternatives, at the same time as needing to make definite decisions and recommendations one way or the other.

There are occasions, in response to questions from patients or from students as to causes, in complex cases, where single aetiology of large effect has been excluded, and the picture looks more like multiple aetiology of small effect, it is as correct as anything else to say:'it is a complex biopsychosocial picture'. This move is by all means somewhat vague and hand-waving, connected to the criticism of the biopsychosocial model reviewed in the first chapter, that it is vague and too often used for unhelpful hand-waving. Engel's model has stood ready to accommodate emerging findings of biopsychosocial complexity, and being so accommodating has made it hard to capture in a few words except vaguely. However, complexity and uncertainty have come from the science; they are not peculiar features of a model—no point blaming the messenger. And, in fairness to the biopsychosocial model, the generalised single primary cause models are the same—vague hand-waving to everything being biological/biomedical, or else all psychological, or social. The science of the past few decades has all but ruled out these single primary cause general models, and endorsed the broader biopsychosocial approach. The broader approach is also able to be more discriminating, more empirically based than the previous generalised single factor models. Biological, psychological and social factors may be involved in specific health conditions, at specific stages, but whether they are or not, and in what degree, is not known in advance, but only by doing the science.

4.4 Compare and Contrast Physical and Mental Health Conditions

Psychiatry and 'The Rest of Medicine'

Psychiatry is obviously psychological, at first glance, but also obviously social, at second glance, while biological to a degree, while the rest of medicine—according to the biomedical model—manages well enough with the biological only. In this sense, the question of psychiatry's relation to 'the rest of medicine' stands proxy for the rationale and validity of the biopsychosocial model—and vice versa. In fact, Engel chose just this issue as the starting place for his 1977 paper; he turned on its head the aspiration for psychiatry to emulate the rest of medicine, recommending the opposite: make the rest of medicine more like psychiatry—more psychosocial, not biological only [4] (p. 129).

On the other hand, as we noted at the beginning of the first chapter (under the heading "The Presumed 'Overarching Framework'"), the 'rest of medicine' is not one thing, and the various medical specialities differ in their relative involvement with biological, psychological and social factors. Primary care (also known as general medical practice, or family medicine) is much involved with the psychosocial, as is public health, and palliative care, as well as many aspects of care on acute medical wards. In this sense, the contrast is not so much between psychiatry with the rest of medicine, but between psychiatry along with many other areas of medicine, contrasted with biomedicine. Taking these considerations things into account much qualifies the idea that psychiatry is so different because of its involvement with the psychosocial. Nevertheless, psychiatry can still be regarded as the odd one out compared with 'the rest of medicine', for reasons that go much deeper than detailed and discriminating considerations of the above sort about varying degrees of involvement with the psychosocial.

The Difference Is Deeply Theorised and Institutionalised

The perceived difference between mental and physical health conditions and healthcare is underpinned by the great historical dichotomies outlined in the first chapter, Sect. 1.3 (under the heading "Prejudicial Theory: Physicalism, Reductionism, Dualism"): mind/body dualism, and the separation of the social and moral sciences from the natural sciences. Thomas Szasz's highly influential 1960s critique of psychiatry [54] relied on these dichotomies. But worse, the two sides of the dichotomies were not equally balanced in respect of scientific validity, especially in connection with determining causes and interventions—matters fundamental to medicine. Rather, against the background of physicalist reductionism, which underpinned the dichotomies, as reviewed in Sect. 2.2, while physical health conditions involved recognised causes and effects, researchable and manageable by proper biological/biomedical science, mental disorders were something else altogether, barely recognisable let alone theorised, and psychiatry along with them.

Built on top of the historical dichotomies in deep theory are the reinforcing, maintaining effects of having organised the whole of healthcare training and delivery around physical health problems on one side of the road and mental health problems on the other. On one side, biomedicine performs best with biological mechanisms in physical diseases, and psychosocial involvement, if any, is out of scope. On the other side, theoretical or practical preoccupation with 'mental abnormalities' such as delusions and other hard to understand mental states and behaviour tends to neglect somatic signs and symptoms, and does not bring into focus people as a whole and their social circumstances. The dichotomy between mental and physical health conditions is historically theorised and currently institutionalised and practised.

The Biopsychosocial Model Highlights Similarities

There are several reasons why the picture is changing however. Mental health conditions are more evident, linked to increasing public awareness and efforts to decrease stigma, and the extent of associated activity impairments such as days lost to work is better understood and increasingly recognised as comparable with those in physical health conditions. It is increasingly recognised that physical and mental health problems often co-occur, complicating each other, and therefore also complicating our healthcare system, given that it is currently organised on the basis of separating them out, along with the clinical expertise for managing them. And as regards aetiology, public health and prevention, recent epidemiology suggests that the two kinds of health problem can share aetiological risk factors, possibly implicating shared mechanisms. These social and scientific developments change policy, as for example in the UK NHS policy paper 'No health without mental health' [55]. In this section, we review these issues in more detail, with reference to the biopsychosocial theory and science set out in previous chapters.

Considering aetiology, we noted in the first chapter, Sect. 1.2, the emerging epidemiological evidence that implicates psychosocial as well as biological risk factors including genetic for many physical health conditions. It also suggests that some risks of all sorts are shared between some physical health conditions and some mental health conditions; it is not the case that risk factors divide neatly into those to physical health on the one hand and those to mental health on the other. Drilling into hypothesised mechanisms, we saw in section Stress as a Biopsychosocial

Causal Mechanism that chronic stress and its biological effects are commonly implicated in the aetiology of many physical and mental health conditions. Again, it is not the case that pathogenic mechanisms neatly divide between those for physical health conditions and those for mental health conditions. As corollary, preventative strategies and technologies, for many physical and mental health conditions, overlap. Public health does not have two unconnected tasks, one for physical health promotion and another for mental health promotion.

Post onset, especially for the long-term conditions, also considered in Sect. 1.2 under the heading "Emerging Evidence of Psychosocial Causation", psychosocial factors affect biomedical management, in matters such as access and collaboration over management plan, for example ongoing medication; as well as affecting psychological adjustment and quality of social life. These diverse psychosocial issues coincide or at least overlap for both physical health and mental health long term conditions. We went on to note the connected finding that physical health problems raise risk for mental health problems and vice versa. The causal pathways are diverse, but include such as chronic physical ill-health imposes activity restrictions and loss of amenity, and pain, all of which raise risk of high anxiety and low mood; mental health chronic conditions can be associated with risk factors for physical health problems, such as social exclusion, poor diet, smoking, and higher thresholds for medical attention to physical health problems. The picture that emerges, therefore, is not that of patients with physical health problems, and an entirely different set of patients with mental health problems. All these considerations—regarding aetiology, adjustment, quality of life, and bidirectional complications—serve to break down the dichotomy between mental health conditions and physical health conditions. They highlight the importance of psychological and social as well as biological factors in health and disease, and they need broad biopsychosocial theory to accommodate them.

The general drift of the biopsychosocial systemic approach—as can be expected from its name—is to view physical and mental health conditions under a unified 'health problem' heading. The core common feature is a substantial negative effect on the person's agency, associated with distress: with worry and fear about their safety and their future and their dependents.

In the broader biopsychosocial picture, the key secondary difference between physical health problems and health problems is that some but not all physical health problems have a biomedically identifiable maintaining cause—a disease process or lesion—while this is probably not the case for mental health problems. This is a critical difference and it stands out most clearly for physical health problems that are biomedically well understood and treatable, in a relatively short timeframe, without therefore impacting on what is presupposed as an otherwise normal life. Cure of infectious disease by antibiotics, surgical interventions that are now routine such as hip replacements and even cardiac surgery, especially where all the psychological and social conditions for access, detection and intervention are in place, and which therefore can be ignored, stand out as triumphs of biomedicine. If we start with the underlying presumption that physical health problems are purely physical—and entirely different from mental health problems—these are the cases we will attend to, and we would tend to neglect the kinds and aspects of physical health problems that don't fit the picture: regarding aetiology, chronic conditions and comorbidities as reviewed briefly above. And, coming from the other direction, the assumption that mental health problems are quite different from physical health problems because exclusively to do with the mind, or the person, is also problematic. For example, some mental health conditions have some response to pharmacotherapy. It is true that psychological therapy is often indicated along with medication for mental health conditions, but equally, as is now being recognised, it is often indicated alongside medical management of physical health conditions [56]. As to mental health conditions, as opposed to physical health conditions, being integral to the personality, the contrast is less marked for long-term conditions of either type, as previously remarked in Sect. 4.2. Also, some mental health conditions such as obsessive-compulsive disorder are typically seen by the person as externally imposed, rather than as integral to themselves. This is probably the rule for mental health conditions rather than the exception. This is a complicated clinical area but the point, in short, is that only for a particular sub-class of mental health conditions is there a strong presumed link with personality, that is, the so-called 'personality disorders'.

Another way of viewing the similarities and differences between mental health conditions and physical health conditions is through the lens of the hypothetical virtual biopsychosocial research framework sketched above (Sect. 4.3). In addition to the specification of biological and neurological systemic functioning, this framework was imagined to include specification of health problems, physical and mental, and to have complete coverage of stages, from risks of onset through to post-onset maintaining causal mechanisms, interventions, and factors affecting adjustment and quality-of-life in long-term conditions. The columns of the grid would include biological, psychological and social factors, and the cells research findings. The upshot of this is that the relative importance of biological compared with psychosocial factors would be most marked between mental and some physical health problems at just one—albeit very important—point, namely post-onset maintaining causal mechanisms and interventions. For some physical health problems, these would be mainly biological with little psychosocial. But for all other stages: aetiological pathways to onset, and post-onset adjustment and quality-of-life, the pattern of relative weights of biological, psychological and social would be evened out and would certainly not be all biological for all physical health problems, and all psychological and social for mental health problems.

4.5 Locating the Biopsychosocial Model

We noted in the first chapter that the biopsychosocial model has been charged with *vagueness* in the clinic, as well as vagueness as a scientific theory and as a 'model'. It is true that Engel wrote his 1980 paper [5] on clinical application of the model, giving rise to the reasonable inference that the biopsychosocial model was a guide to clinical practice. However, as we went on to note in Sect. 1.2, there have been many developments in the intervening decades with more direct relevance to scientific content and guiding clinical practice. There have been new research programmes to investigate the causes of diseases and disease mechanisms, and technologies for prevention, early detection and treatment. These, in turn, have led to treatment guidelines for specific conditions at specific stages, to the whole apparatus of evidence-based clinical care, to be used alongside a thorough assessment of the individual case. The point is simply that, given all this basic and clinical science of the last few decades, the biopsychosocial model cannot usefully be regarded as some additional statement of the science or as a tool to guide clinical decision-making. It is true the model advises us to keep one's mind open to the range of biopsychosocial factors, but the treatment guidelines and the science behind them already now say this, if applicable, and we don't need a general model to repeat the fact—especially not to repeat it vaguely instead of paying close attention to the science of specific conditions and stages.

While this may be a solution for the biopsychosocial model of the vagueness problem, it works only, as we noted in section "So What's the Point of a 'General Model'?", by raising the more fundamental question: what is the point of having a general model at all? We then located the task of the general model as defining biopsychosocial ontology and causation, in Sect. 1.3, noting the special need for this because of the deeply entrenched assumptions of physicalism, dualism and reductionism that have been so influential in the development of the life and human sciences. With these assumptions, only physical properties and causation appear real, while the mind is a non-causal epiphenomena, and social organisation and processes can hardly be comprehended at all. In short, the scientific and philosophical back story is more or less entirely antithetical to theorising biopsychosocial ontology and interactions. Hence the need for a new general theory for this purpose. We pursued this, tracking the science, in Chapters 2 and 3.

In Chapter 2 on biology we used the approach especially suited for the present purpose that relates biological processes to physics. Life forms do extraordinary things with energy, holding up the general direction of the second law of thermodynamics, for a while, the key being control by genetic code, essentially prone to error, to doing it differently, making space for evolutionary diversification. The key ontological shift compared with physicalism is away from few primary physical qualities and laws, variations on the theme of energy and energy conservation, towards multiplicity and diversity of dynamical forms with their own distinctive principles of change and causal interaction, all however retaining consistency with the physics of the matter. The corresponding key epistemological shifts are from generality to specificity, simplicity to complexity, and from knowledge of inviolable facts to active knowing, something more like 'trial and error'. Moving on from biology, the psychological and the social were considered in Chapter 3. The primary concept of the psychological is identified as agency. This connotes altogether: causation, in the sense of regulatory control, authorship, individual differences, and self-determination. Agency is thoroughly biological: it is embodied, and accordingly has to secure the conditions necessary for biological life, specifically those related to maintaining appropriate energy differentials. At the same time, agency for us social beings needs recognition in the social group, and generally assumes a socio-political dimension, connoted by the related concept of autonomy. The primary function of the social is identified in the model as the regulatory control of the distribution of resources necessary for biological life, but also of resources and opportunities for psychological development and cultivation of agency.

In this biopsychosocial theory, concepts of health and disease appear in prototypical form at the beginning, in the differences between survival and non-survival of biological organisms, between a biological system's working or breaking down. The basic facts of biological health and disease carry through into the biopsychosocial whole, being joined by concepts of psychological health and ill-health, related to agency, and concepts of psychosocial health and disadvantage, marked by exclusion from social relationships, resources and opportunities. Causal pathways run within and between all these systems and the many subsystems that serve them, in health and ill-health. The exact pathways and the size of effects vary with the health condition, its stage, and the challenges it presents to the person as agent.

As well as major developments in the basic and clinical sciences since Engel's original papers, there have been other major developments in dedicated models of health and disease and clinical practice. Three such have been mentioned so far in this chapter, Sect. 4.2: the social model of disability, which contests attribution of cause of activity limitations to the person rather than to the ill-resourced, socially excluding environment; the model of patient-centred care, which locates the person as patient, their aims and values, at the centre of healthcare, and the Recovery model, which theorises the need of the person with a chronic health condition to recover their life notwithstanding. These dedicated models emphasise specific important aspects of healthcare that broadly relate to individual differences, the person, the broader social and political context, and managing with chronic conditions—typically with explicit contrast with a perceived simple and over-simple 'medical model', with its focus on biological disease processes in the individual. In this sense, these models have taken up challenges and tasks of the sort that Engel identified, but with more elaboration, depth and detail than the biopsychosocial model itself.

As proposed here, biopsychosocial theory and the biopsychosocial model define the conceptual foundations of a new approach to health, disease and healthcare, one that responds to the accumulating evidence implicating many and diverse processes of kinds indicated by the name, and more besides, particularly the physics and chemistry of our bodies and the environment, at one end, and social and economic policy at the other. It is more general than the science of specifics, or single disciplines, or dedicated models of clinical care. It is more like a view of human nature, based in the current science, one that includes propensity to health and disease. As a view of human nature and its vulnerabilities, the biopsychosocial model is comparable to the biomedical model. The biomedical model has two versions however: the old version, running to approximately mid-twentieth century, assuming, as Engel saw, physicalist reductionism and dualism, the other brand new and going from strength to strength since, at the cutting edge of reconstructing the relationship between biology, physics and chemistry, and articulating new models involving not only the inviolable physics and chemistry of energy, but also vulnerable forms regulated to ends. The new research programmes have advanced biomedicine, but at a conceptual level they open up worlds beyond the biological to include the psychological and the social. This conceptual opening up is of huge importance given that the conceptual foundations of health science and healthcare need to be able to comprehend and respond to all the new findings on psychosocial factors that have been accumulating over the past few decades, on the social determinants of health, the effectiveness of psychological and social treatments, and the increasing prevalence of long-term health conditions.

Biopsychosocial theory, incorporating the psychosocial and the political, also involves morality. The biopsychosocial model of health and disease has conceptual connections with bioethics. This is a contrast with the biomedical model, in either its old or new forms. To the extent that the biomedical model embraced physicalist reductionism, it was not entitled to any normative concepts, not even the difference between health and disease, and definitely not morals. Normativity has no place in physics and chemistry. The new biomedical model that invokes regulatory control mechanisms has normativity, but so far restricted to internal somatic systems and does not yet comprehend the whole human being as an agent in the interpersonal, socio-political world. To have this reach, the biopsychosocial model is required, and the term 'bioethics' could be expanded to 'biopsychosocial ethics'. At the foundational level, all normativity is interconnected. The 4 principles of bioethics laid out by Beauchamp and Childress [57] employ terms and relations that are foundational in biopsychosocial theory: autonomy of the person, harm and benefits to the person, social distribution of resources. The biopsychosocial theory does not resolve ethical disputes but indicates their terms and the friction points where they arise. Biological health, psychological health, autonomous exercise of agency and values, social provision of resources necessary for these things—are all goods from our point of view as biopsychosocial beings, but they can be hard to achieve together since they can come into conflict one with one another. The individual may come into conflict with family, clinicians or the law, over what is good for them; what is in the interests of the individual may conflict with what is in the interests of the community; attribution of 'illness' or 'disability' may have benefits in terms of access to healthcare and support, but it downgrades recognition of autonomy, with potential for harm; provision of resources can conflict with promoting agency; equal distribution of resources competes with individual and group interests. And there are boundary issues, for example as to when biological life becomes psychological life with moral value protected by law, or as to when psychological life has come to an end in severe brain damage while the biology continues. Biopsychosocial theory cannot resolve these many kinds of moral dilemmas, but their terms and the potential for conflicts over priorities and boundaries appear at its foundations.

References

1. Jaspers, K. (1962). *Allgemeine pychopathologie* [General psychopathology] (J. Hoenig, M. W. Hamilton, trans.). Manchester: Manchester University Press. (Original work published 1913).
2. Shakespeare, T. (2006). The social model of disability. In L. J. Davies (Ed.), *The disability studies reader* (2nd ed., pp. 197–204). New York & Oxford: Routledge.
3. Oliver, M. (2013). The social model of disability: Thirty years on. *Disability & Society, 28*(7), 1024–1026. https://doi.org/10.1080/09687599.2013.818773.
4. Engel, G. L. (1977). The need for a new medical model: A challenge for biomedicine. *Science, 196*(4286), 129–136.
5. Engel, G. L. (1980). The clinical application of the biopsychosocial model. *American Journal of Psychiatry, 137*(5), 535–544.
6. Brody, H. (1999). The biopsychosocial model, patient-centered care, and culturally sensitive practice. *The Journal of Family Practice, 48*(8), 585–587.
7. Creed, F. (2005). Are the patient-centred and biopsychosocial approaches compatible. In P. D. White (Ed.), *Biopsychosocial medicine: An integrated approach to understanding illness* (pp. 187–199). New York: Oxford University Press.

8. Smith, R. C., Fortin, A. H., Dwamena, F., & Frankel, R. M. (2013). An evidence-based patient-centered method makes the biopsychosocial model scientific. *Patient Education and Counseling, 91*(3), 265–270. https://doi.org/10.1016/j.pec.2012.12.010.
9. Evers, A. W. M., Gieler, U., Hasenbring, M. I., & van Middendorp, H. (2014). Incorporating biopsychosocial characteristics into personalized healthcare: A clinical approach. *Psychotherapy and Psychosomatics, 83*(3), 148–157. https://doi.org/10.1159/000358309.
10. Davidson, L., & Strauss, J. S. (1995). Beyond the biopsychosocial model: Integrating disorder, health, and recovery. *Psychiatry, 58*(1), 44–55.
11. Frese, F. J., III, Stanley, J., Kress, K., & Vogel-Scibilia, S. (2001). Integrating evidence-based practices and the recovery model. *Psychiatric Services, 52*(11), 1462–1468.
12. Slade, M. (2009). *Personal recovery and mental illness: A guide for mental health professionals.* Cambridge: Cambridge University Press.
13. Bennett, B., Breeze, J., & Neilson, T. (2014). Applying the recovery model to physical rehabilitation. *Nursing Standard, 28*(23), 37–43.
14. Boorse, C. (1975). On the distinction between disease and illness. *Philosophy & Public Affairs, 5*(1), 49–68.
15. Boyd, K. M. (2000). Disease, illness, sickness, health, healing and wholeness: Exploring some elusive concepts. *Med Humanit, 26*(1), 9–17.
16. Osler, W. (2009). *Aequanimitas and other addresses.* San Francisco, CA: Internet Archive (Original work published 1904).
17. Huber, M., Knottnerus, J. A., Green, L., Horst, H., Jadad, A. R., Kromhout, D., et al. (2011). How should we define health? *BMJ, 343.* [https://doi.org/10.1136/bmj.d4163].
18. Wittgenstein, L. (1953). *Philosophical Investigations.* (G. E. M. Anscombe, Trans.). Oxford: Blackwell.
19. Hardcastle, V. G. (1999). *The myth of pain.* Cambridge, MA: The MIT Press.
20. Bourke, J. (2014). *The story of pain: From prayer to painkillers.* Oxford: Oxford University Press.
21. Melzack, R., & Wall, P. (1965). Pain mechanisms: A new theory. *Science, 150*(3699), 971–979. https://doi.org/10.1126/science.150.3699.971.
22. Fields, H. L. (2007). Setting the stage for pain: Allegorical tales from neuroscience. In S. Coakley & K. K. Shelemay (Eds.), *Pain and its transformations: The interface of biology and culture* (pp. 36–61). Cambridge, MA: Harvard University Press.
23. Quartana, P. J., Campbell, C. M., & Edwards, R. R. (2009). Pain catastrophizing: A critical review. *Expert Review of Neurotherapeutics, 9*(5), 745–758. https://doi.org/10.1586/ern.09.34.
24. Craig, K. D. (2009). The social communication model of pain. *Canadian Psychology, 50*(1), 22–32.

25. Williams, A. C. C. (2002). Facial expression of pain: An evolutionary account. *Behavioral and Brain Sciences, 25*(4), 439–455.
26. Hales, C. N., & Barker, D. J. P. (2001). The thrifty phenotype hypothesis: Type 2 diabetes. *British Medical Bulletin, 60*(1), 5–20.
27. Patterson, G. R., DeBaryshe, B. D., & Ramsey, E. (1989). A developmental perspective on antisocial behavior. *American Psychologist, 44*(2), 329–335.
28. Patterson, G. R. (1982). *Coercive family process.* Eugene, OR: Castalia.
29. Russo, F., & Williamson, J. (2007). Interpreting causality in the health sciences. *International Studies in the Philosophy of Science, 21*(2), 157–170. https://doi.org/10.1080/02698590701498084.
30. Illari, P. M., & Williamson, J. (2011). Mechanisms are real and local. In P. M. Illari, F. Russo, & J. Williamson (Eds.), *Causality in the sciences* (pp. 818–844). Oxford: Oxford University Press.
31. Machamer, P., Darden, l., & Craver, C. F. (2000). Thinking about Mechanisms. *Philosophy of Science, 67*(1), 1–25.
32. Glennan, S. (2002). Rethinking mechanistic explanation. *Philosophy of Science, 69*(S3), S342–S353.
33. Kincaid, H. (2011). Causal modelling, mechanism, and probability in epidemiology. In P. M. Illari, F. Russo, & J. Williamson (Eds.), *Causality in the sciences* (pp. 70–90). Oxford: Oxford University Press.
34. Kendler, K. S., & Campbell, J. (2009). Interventionist causal models in psychiatry: Repositioning the mind-body problem. *Psychological Medicine, 39*(6), 881–887. https://doi.org/10.1017/S0033291708004467.
35. Broadbent, A. (2011). Inferring causation in epidemiology: Mechanisms, black boxes and contrasts. In P. M. Illari, F. Russo, & J. Williamson (Eds.), *Causality in the sciences* (pp. 45–69). Oxford: Oxford University Press.
36. Leuridan, B., & Weber, E. (2011). The IARC and mechanistic evidence. In P. M. Illari, F. Russo, & J. Williamson (Eds.), *Causality in the sciences* (pp. 91–109). Oxford: Oxford University Press.
37. Steptoe, A. (2005). Remediable or preventable psychological factors in the aetiology and prognosis of medical disorders. In P. White (Ed.), *Biopsychosocial medicine* (pp. 59–75). Oxford: Oxford University Press.
38. Lightman, S. (2005). Can neurobiology explain the relationship between stress and disease. In P. White (Ed.), *Biopsychosocial medicine* (pp. 103–111). Oxford: Oxford University Press.
39. Buric, I., Farias, M., Jong, J., Mee, C., & Brazil, I. A. (2017). What is the molecular signature of mind–body interventions? A systematic review of gene expression changes induced by meditation and related practices. *Frontiers in Immunology, 8*(670). https://doi.org/10.3389/fimmu.2017.00670.
40. Slavich, G. M., & Irwin, M. R. (2014). From stress to inflammation and major depressive disorder: A social signal transduction theory of depression. *Psychological Bulletin, 140*(3), 774–815.

41. Tawakol, A., Ishai, A., Takx, R. A. P., Figueroa, A. L., Ali, A., Kaiser, Y., et al. (2017). Relation between resting amygdalar activity and cardiovascular events: A longitudinal and cohort study. *The Lancet, 389*(10071), 834–845.
42. Rotter, J. B. (1966). Generalized expectancies for internal versus external control of reinforcement. *Psychological Monographs: General and Applied, 80*(1), 1–28.
43. Seligman, M. E. P. (1972). Learned helplessness. *Annual Review of Medicine, 23*(1), 407–412.
44. Lazarus, R. S. (1999). *Stress and emotion: A new synthesis.* London: Free Association Books.
45. Insel, T., Cuthbert, B., Garvey, M., Heinssen, R., Pine, D. S., Quinn, K., et al. (2010). Research domain criteria (RDoC): Toward a new classification framework for research on mental disorders. *American Journal of Psychiatry, 167*(7), 748–751.
46. Cuthbert, B. N. (2014). The RDoC framework: Facilitating transition from ICD/DSM to dimensional approaches that integrate neuroscience and psychopathology. *World Psychiatry, 13*(1), 28–35.
47. Wakefield, J. C. (2014). Wittgenstein's nightmare: Why the RDoC grid needs a conceptual dimension. *World Psychiatry, 13*(1), 38–40.
48. Phillips, M. R. (2014). Will RDoC hasten the decline of America's global leadership role in mental health? *World Psychiatry, 13*(1), 40–41.
49. Bolton, D. (2017). Clinical significance, disability and biomarkers: Shifts in thinking between DSM-4 and DSM-5. In K. Kendler, & J. Parnas (Eds.), *Philosophical Issues in Psychiatry IV. Psychiatric Nosology* (pp. 8–16). Oxford: Oxford University Press.
50. Kelly, M. P., Stewart, E., Morgan, A., Killoran, A., Fischer, A., Threlfall, A., et al. (2009). A conceptual framework for public health: NICE's emerging approach. *Public Health, 123*(1), e14–e20. https://doi.org/10.1016/j.puhe.2008.10.031.
51. Evidence-Based Medicine Working Group. (1992). Evidence-based medicine. A new approach to teaching the practice of medicine. *Journal of the American Medical Association, 268*(17), 2420.
52. Greenhalgh, T., Howick, J., & Maskrey, N. (2014). Evidence based medicine: A movement in crisis? *British Medical Journal, 348,* g3725.
53. Bolton, D. (2008). The epistemology of randomized, controlled trials and application in psychiatry. *Philosophy, Psychiatry & Psychology, 15*(2), 159–165.
54. Szasz, T. (1961). *The myth of mental illness.* New York: Harper and Row.
55. HM Government. (2011). No health without mental health: A cross-government mental health outcomes strategy for people of all ages. London, UK: Department of Health. https://www.gov.uk/government/publications/no-health-without-mental-health-a-cross-government-mental-health-outcomes-strategy-for-people-of-all-ages-a-call-to-action.

56. NHS England, & NHS Improvement. (2018). The Improving Access to Psychological Therapies (IAPT) pathway for people with long-term physical health conditions and medically unexplained symptoms. https://www.england.nhs.uk/publication/the-improving-access-to-psychological-therapies-iapt-pathway-for-people-with-long-term-physical-health-conditions-and-medically-unexplained-symptoms/.
57. Beauchamp, T. L., & Childress, J. F. (2012). *Principles of biomedical ethics* (7th ed.). New York: Oxford University Press.

Index

D. Bolton and G. Gillett, *The Biopsychosocial Model of Health and Disease*,
https://doi.org/10.1007/978-3-030-11899-0

www.ingramcontent.com/pod-product-compliance
Lightning Source LLC
LaVergne TN
LVHW082236200926
848484LV00008B/2363